Medical Sociology and Old Age

Towards a sociology of health in later life

Paul Higgs and Ian Rees Jones

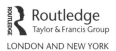

Routledge
Taylor & Francis Group

LONDON AND NEW YORK

First published 2009
by Routledge
2 Park Square, Milton Park, Abingdon, Oxon OX14 4RN

Simultaneously published in the USA and Canada
by Routledge
270 Madison Avenue, New York, NY 10016

Routledge is an imprint of the Taylor & Francis Group, an informa business

© 2009 Paul Higgs and Ian Rees Jones

Typeset in Sabon by
Taylor & Francis Books
Printed and bound in Great Britain by
TJ International Ltd, Padstow Cornwall

British Library Cataloguing in Publication Data
A catalogue record for this book is available from the British Library

Library of Congress Cataloging in Publication Data
Higgs, Paul.
    Medical sociology and old age : towards a sociology of health in later life /
Paul Higgs and Ian Rees Jones.
        p. cm. – (Critical studies in health and society)
    Includes bibliographical references.
    1. Older people–Health and hygiene–Social aspects. 2. Social medicine. I.
Jones, Ian Rees. II. Title. III. Series.
    [DNLM: 1. Aged. 2. Geriatrics. 3. Sociology, Medical. WT 30 H637m 2008]
    RA564.8.H54 2008
362.198'97–dc22   2008018379

ISBN 978-0-415-39855-8 (hbk)   *1005559860*
ISBN 978-0-415-39860-2 (pbk)
ISBN 978-0-203-88872-8 (ebk)

Contents

Medical Sociology and Old Age

As populations throughout the world grow older, the health of older people becomes more and more important for policy makers and the public alike. This book reflects on how our understanding and experience of health at later ages interacts with social and bio-medical developments.

The nature of health in later life has conventionally been studied fromtwo perspectives. Medical sociologists have focused on the failing body, chronic illness, infirmity and mortality, while social gerontologists on the other hand have focused on the epidemiology of old age and health and social policy. By examining these perspectives, Higgs and Jones show how both standpoints have a restricted sense of contemporary ageing which has prevented an understanding of the way in which health in later life has changed. In the book, the authors point out that the current debates on longevity and disability are being transformed by the emergence of a fitter and healthier older population. This third age – where fitness and participation are valorised – leads to the increasing salience of issues such as bodily control, age-denial and anti-ageing medicine. By discussing the key issue of old age versus ageing, the authors examine the prospect of a new sociology – a sociology of health in later life.

Medical Sociology and Old Age is essential reading for all students and researchers of medical sociology and gerontology and for anyone concerned with the challenge of ageing populations in the twenty-first century.

Paul Higgs is Professor of the Sociology of Ageing at University College London.

Ian Rees Jones is Professor of Sociology of Health at Bangor University, Wales.

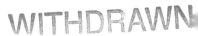

Critical Studies in Health and Society
Series Editors: Simon J. Williams & Gillian Bendelow

This major new international book series takes a critical look at health in a rapidly changing social world. The series includes theoretically sophisticated and empirically informed contributions on cutting-edge issues from leading figures within the sociology of health and allied disciplines and domains. Other titles in the series include:

Contesting Psychiatry
Social movements in mental health
Nick Crossley

Lifestyle in Medicine
Gary Easthope and Emily Hansen

Medical Sociology and Old Age
Towards a sociology of health in later life
Paul Higgs and Ian Rees Jones

Emotional Labour in Health Care
The unmanaged heart of nursing
Catherine Theodosius

Globalisation, Markets and Healthcare Policy
Redrawing the patient as consumer
Jonathan Tritter, Meri Koivusalo and Eeva Ollila

Written in a lively, accessible and engaging style, with many thought-provoking insights, the series will cater to a truly interdisciplinary audience of researchers, professionals, practitioners and policy makers with an interest in health and social change.

Those interested in submitting proposals for single or co-authored, edited or co-edited volumes should contact the series editors, Simon J. Williams (s.j.williams @warwick.ac.uk) and Gillian Bendelow (g.a.bendelow@sussex.ac.uk).

Preface

The idea for this book was in part motivated by the fact that both of us worked in fields that straddled the subject areas of medical sociology and social gerontology. While we felt that there were many overlaps between what we were doing in both fields, it became more and more clear that we were in fact dealing with two separate worlds, each with their own literatures and pre-occupations. What was striking was that with a few notable exceptions such as Margot Jeffreys and Mike Bury there were few who seemed to be aware of the material that existed on either side of the 'divide'. Consequently this book arose out of a need to try to address this gap as much for ourselves as for others undoubtedly dealing with the same issues.

A further motivation came from the fact that not only was ageing becoming a larger and larger issue for social policy (Esping-Andersen 2002), but it was also affecting the discussion about the provision of health services for the population as a whole as can be seen in the work surrounding the Wanless Report (Wanless 2001). A pleasing consequence of this rise to prominence of ageing in the wider world was that our work on older people and later life became more interesting to colleagues who had previously seen it as a bit of an intellectual and research backwater. The attention, however, also demonstrated that many of the assumptions that were held about ageing by quite a few social scientists were limited in their understanding of contemporary ageing. We were also aware that many of these assumptions had, in part, resulted from much of the work that researchers in ageing such as us had been responsible for. This was all the more problematic because we were also aware of how the terrain of ageing was changing and how it necessitated different conceptual tools and approaches. Indeed, the changes in the nature of old age, the impact of consumerism and technology as well as the role of generation all indicated that an engagement with a more sociologically informed set of ideas was necessary. Certainly we are not the first to come to this conclusion. Bryan Turner in his *The New Medical Sociology* (Turner 2004) points out the importance of ageing when trying to understand the changing nature of health and illness in the twenty-first century. He links the ageing body around impairment and disability, and points out the importance of time and context in understanding the relationship between age and health. However, in general we have found that few have as yet got beyond seeing ageing as a residual category. In both Williams and Bendelow (1998) and Crossley (2001), volumes on the lived body and the social body respectively, there is little or no engagement with the issue of ageing embodiment (although Simon Williams rectifies this in a later work, see Williams, 2003) and it will be interesting to see if revised versions of standard medical sociology textbooks will devote more space to the issue in the future. It is also not the case that writers in the mainstream of the discipline are any more aware of the issues of ageing and later life. Ageing itself is generally seen to be outside the purview of most general socio-logical texts on social structure – the omission being generally un-noticed and not seen as needing rectification. Harriet Bradley (1996) in her *Fractured Identities: Changing Patterns of Inequality* explicitly points this out by calling her chapter 'Age: The neglected dimension of stratification'. The fact that this book is over a decade old and there has been little subsequent engagement suggests that age is still a neglected dimension within sociology.

Our desire in writing this book was therefore to help rectify this anomaly especially as the issues of ageing in a somatic society not only presented many opportunities to develop medical sociology but also made an engagement with the issues thrown up by later life essential for the continuing relevance of the sub-discipline. However, if coming to grips with an ageing society is important for medical sociology, likewise understanding how it has changed is also crucial for the continuing development of social gerontology. While there have been many research initiatives around old age in the UK, social gerontology has remained a relatively weak and peripheral field of study. There are no undergraduate programmes in gerontology and no funding organisations with the power of the US National Institutes of Aging organising research priorities on later life. Whereas in the US research has been focused on determinants of successful or productive ageing, the focus in Britain has been more around the needs of social and health policy with an emphasis on the 'structured dependency' of older people. The landmark studies in British social gerontology, Townsend's *The Last Refuge* (Townsend 1962) and *Family Life of Older People* (1957) continue to set a framework for studying later life that centres on marginalisation of older people by state and public institutions.

In the USA, the emphasis on 'successful ageing' reflected the dominance of medical and psychological paradigms on research trajectories. Indeed, much of the work that is published in gerontological journals continues to adopt either an epidemiological or psychological rather than sociological approach to issues of health. However, this does not mean that there has been no theoretical elaboration of a sociology of ageing (Riley, Johnson and Foner 1972), but it has been dominated by various attempts to establish a political economy approach to ageing (Estes, Linkins and Binney 1996). In both countries a key aspect of what has now come to be identified as 'critical gerontology' has been a critique of the presentation of old age as an economic and social burden while at the same time being the source of profits for managed care and medical insurance companies (Estes 2001). In this there is little discussion of how health and disability interact, other than by reference to the social policies that situate it.

While critical gerontology has made a number of important and telling points with regard to the construction of old age by, and through, the needs of corporate medical industrial complexes (Estes 1979), and has expanded its ambit to discussions of identity, neo-liberalism and globalisation, it still seems unable to abandon its connections to social policy and 1970s Marxism. Indeed, Green (1993) suggests that social gerontology is an 'incoherent domain of theory' applied to both individual and cohort ageing. This hampers it in its attempts to develop explanations for the rapid changes to later life experienced in recent years. As the geriatrician Raymond Tallis points out, there appears to be incongruence between the concerns of social gerontology and the fact that the rapid increases in life expectancy and quality of life at later ages are strongly related to advances in medical science and preventative techniques:

> Why is there such a 'miserabilist' response to the increases we've seen in life expectancy in rich countries? The evidence is that the levels of ill-health and disability in older people at any given age

are falling – a tribute to the effectiveness of health promotion, preventive medicine and acute medical care. Old people are living not only longer but also in better nick.

(Tallis 2005)

It is not only in terms of the reaction to changes in longevity and health that the position is problematic. There also seems to be hostility to engaging with many of the other complex changes that have occurred to ageing which do not place the old in a dependent position. The rise of a cultural gerontology has found itself sometimes at odds with the conventional accounts adopted by those social gerontologists influenced by critical gerontology (Walker 2005). As a result, making a case for a different approach to the study of *health* in later life was also one of the motivations for writing this book, allowing as it did the opportunity to present a whole number of issues, both theoretical and contextual, in a different light.

In writing this book we are not claiming to provide an exhaustive overview of either the medical sociology of later life or of social gerontology. We are aware that there are many writers and pieces of research that we have not covered or given enough space to. We are also aware that we are providing a prismatic view of the areas we are covering and that maybe some will say that the truth lies somewhere in between. That we can accept. What this book is written to provoke, however, is a discussion about how later life and health need to be understood in the context of social change.

1 Medical sociology and old age

Introduction

There is a widespread consensus that we are living in an age of demographic transition where the challenges of ageing populations in Europe and North America will lead to major problems in the provision of healthcare and in the organisation of social policy (Gee 2000). Not only are individuals living longer but they are also becoming an ever larger proportion of the population when viewed against the size of younger age groups. Generational conflict over resources has long been predicted and the 'grey timebomb' seems to be ticking away (Thomson 1989, Myles 2002). Bryan Turner (2000) is not alone when he sees 'the greying of the west' as a metaphor for the way in which demographic and epidemiological transitions of the twentieth century have combined with increasing affluence to change the landscape of illness in advanced societies. The scene therefore seems to be set for disaster. However, this transition to an older population is not simply a predictable outcome of age-related decline. There is much more to the nature of contemporary ageing than can be simply read off from population statistics. What is emerging is the culmination of long-term demographic trends in the context of distinctly new circumstances. The eminent bio-gerontologist Tom Kirkwood ended his first Reith lecture in 2000 on the 'End of Age' by stating:

> New scientific understanding means that we can never think of ageing in the same way again. We are at the end of the old 'old age'. We know that we will all die one day, but this day is being pushed back further and further. Our longer lives are carrying us into new territory for which we need to plan and prepare ourselves.

We cannot afford to be complacent. If we ignore the implications of the longevity revolution and fail to plan for the radically different world that will soon surround us, then crisis will be upon us and our bright dreams of a brave old world will surely fade and die.

(Kirkwood 2001: 17)

The seeming contradiction between a world growing older and Kirkwood's argument that today's ageing population represent a dramatic defiance of Nature is at the heart of why we need to go beyond the consensus and view ageing in a different light. It is not that attention has not been paid to these developments. Indeed, policy makers are very interested in what might be occurring in a host of different policy areas and on both sides of the Atlantic (Aaron, Shoven and Friedman 1999; House of Lords 2005; Pensions Commission 2005; Wanless 2001). What is missing, however, is a more radical re-examination of how these changes impact on the lives of older people themselves, particularly in those social science disciplines where these changes might be most noticeable and have the greatest impact. Both medical sociology and social gerontology are approaches that have much to say about the changing nature of both health and ageing, however they have not said much about these changes. In part this may be the result of long established disciplinary foci which channel energy into specific pathways and away from topics that seem outside of their purview. It is the argument of this book that it is a conundrum that medical sociology has underplayed the issue of ageing within the mainstream of its thinking while at the same time social gerontology has, with a few notable exceptions, avoided a direct engagement with the knowledge bases of medical sociology. This is true even where the health of older people is directly addressed. In addition, a case can also be made that because of this lack of engagement, novel aspects of this transformation of ageing described above are not given their due significance but rather are interpreted in ways that reintegrate their features into already accepted paradigms.

This chapter charts the relative absence of later life from medical sociology and seeks to take the debate about this major social change forward by suggesting that it is in the social spaces of *second modernity* that a sociology of health in later life will find its new foundations. A sociology of later life needs to address the reality that not only has life expectancy in the UK improved significantly, but that much of post retirement life is lived in relatively good health (Schoeni,

Freedman and Martin 2008). Similarly the issues surrounding the 'somatic society' do not disappear just because an individual is drawing a superannuation pension. The breaking down of the barriers of what constitutes health in society exemplified by terms such as 'healthicization' (Williams 2004) applies as much to the older population as it does to younger groups. By successfully engaging with these changes we would argue that both medical sociology and social gerontology will be more fully able to understand the impact of social changes on ageing and of changes to ageing on the social world of health. This is not just a case of special pleading for a more gerontologically aware medical sociology. Rather it is a recognition that the demographic and epidemiological transitions have more consequences than have been noted to date.

Medical sociology approaching old age

The history of medical sociology has been one of shifting boundaries which have often been reflected in what the sub-discipline chooses to call itself. Conventionally a distinction was made between a sociology *of* medicine and a sociology *in* medicine (Strauss 1957). A further division was also made between medical sociology and the sociology of health and illness, with the latter reflecting the extension of the sociological gaze from medicine to other aspects of healthcare such as the experience of illness. While these terminological disputes may reflect the growth of medical sociology as an area of study it would appear that, with respect to older people at least, old habits die hard and the gaze of medical sociology (or its reformulations) very often ignored or subsumed the older patient into a residual category. To take one example, a recent introductory text book to health sociology (Germov 2005) addresses ageing by linking it to death and dying in a chapter entitled 'Ageing, dying, and death in the twenty-first century'. This is not an isolated case. These gaps were highlighted some time ago by Sara Arber (Arber 1994) but show little sign of disappearing.

While medical sociology has developed branches of research addressing professional interactions, patient experiences and the social epidemiology of health inequalities it has not created a subfield of the sociology of health in later life. Later life has thus tended to be marginalised in specific ways. With respect to the study of inequalities for example, rates of mortality, illness and disability are adjusted for age but until recently there has been a relative lack of interest in the experience of health and illness beyond the age of 'preventable death' at 65. In relation to professional and patient experiences, older patients are often 'interesting' largely to the extent that they are seen to be relatively passive when compared to younger age groups (Lupton 1997). In relation to an area where many of the conditions studied are age-related – chronic illness – there is a notable silence. Indeed, Mike Bury and Jonathan Gabe make reference to this absence in their editors' introduction to *The Sociology of Health and Illness: A Reader* where they comment that:

> much of the chronic illness literature has taken age as a given, referred to often in passing. Much research has been on young or middle aged adults but with little reference to ageing as a process or as a major contextual factor.
>
> (Bury and Gabe 2004: 12)

To understand the lack of attention given to ageing within medical sociology it is necessary to consider the ways in which the sub-discipline developed and how its theoretical and empirical concerns have been moulded in ways that have resulted in ageing being neglected. One possible explanation might be found among medical sociologists themselves. Mike Bury (2000) in his overview of the sociology of health and illness suggests, rather mischievously, that medical sociology's attention to areas such as childbirth, reproduction and middle age may reflect the personal concerns of researchers within the field who have not yet reached later life. However, we would argue that it is more likely that there are stronger structural forces influencing the lack of a sociological gaze on this area.

Medical sociology as a sub-discipline of Sociology emerged in the UK after the Second World War. In the USA the famous chapter 10 of Talcott Parsons' *The Social System* had provided a theoretical basis for medical sociology whereas, as Margot Jeffreys (1997) pointed out, medical sociology in the UK grew out of developments in social medicine in the 1950s and the incorporation of social science into public health research and teaching. At this time Sociology, as a discipline, was underdeveloped within UK academic institutions and within existing departments little attention was given to questions of health and illness. Instead the impetus for sociological work in this area appeared to come from an eclectic mix of economists, social historians, sociologists, anthropologists and statisticians who gradually took on the collective label of medical sociologists. Nevertheless, progress in the field was patchy and resources for secure, long-term posts in medical sociology were not forthcoming. Indeed, frustrated by indifference and sometimes hostility of the medical establishment many medical sociologists (including Jeffreys) moved out of medical departments into mainstream sociology/social science departments where they were able to develop independent research and teaching activities in the field. Matters took a more positive turn following the Royal Commission on Medical Education which reported in 1968 as well as the subsequent General Medical Council recommendation that social aspects of health and illness be a core part of the medical curriculum.

The experiences of researchers like Margot Jeffreys were in marked contrast to those of medical sociologists in the USA. There the development of medical sociology occurred earlier as noted by Bloom (2002), who traces the history of medical sociology as far back as the nineteenth century citing a number of early studies addressing health behaviour and environmental influences on health and illness. In the inter-war period, for example, there were numerous monographs on social pathology tackling such 'social problems' as blindness, deafness, alcoholism and, significantly, old age. However, in Bloom's wide-ranging history it is clear that medical sociology, as a sub-specialty with its own clear social identity, did not fully emerge until after the Second World War. Bloom refers to the influential work of Lawrence J. Henderson, whose structural functionalist approach laid the foundations for Talcott Parsons' seminal work on the sick role. Although Marxist influenced thinkers like Bernhard Stern had opened the door for more critical Marxist accounts of medicine and healthcare the structural functionalism of Parsons became the dominant paradigm for medical sociology in much the same way as it had become the dominant paradigm for sociology as a whole in the USA. This fitted with the post-war optimism and anti-Communist thinking of the time. From 1945 onwards, the pace, volume and intensity of medical sociology research accelerated. A major impetus for the development of medical sociology in the post-war period was funding from the National Institute for Mental Health (NIMH) for investigations addressing the social aspects of mental health problems. Considerable momentum was also gained from support by private foundations, most notably The Commonwealth Fund, The Milbank Memorial Fund, The Rockefeller Foundation and the Russell Sage Foundation. From the late 1950s the creation of the section on Medical Sociology of the American Sociological Association is a key indicator of the rapid growth in the field and marked the creation of a formal professional group within the sociological academy. The focus on social psychiatry declined from the 1970s, as medical sociologists began to move into policy-oriented and health services research. The post-war paradigm however was still heavily influenced by Parsonian functionalism, but from the 1980s the influence of the women's movement and the restructuring of the healthcare industry were both powerful influences on redirecting the focus of medical sociology. Again however, old age was largely ignored in these changes. Indeed, within the American Sociological Association two distinct and separate sections of 'ageing and the life course' and 'medical sociology' came into existence and continue to the current day.

The development of medical sociology was not merely concerned with particular topics of research. Uta Gerhardt in her *Intellectual and Political History of Medical Sociology* identifies four distinct but overlapping theoretical phases for medical sociology (Gerhardt 1989). As noted above the first was Parsons' structural functionalism; the second phase was characterised by the symbolic interactionism inspired by the work of Goffman (1959); the third phase was influenced by phenomenology and the ethnomethodology of Garfinkel (1967); with a fourth phase influenced by Marxism and conflict theory drawing on the work of Zola, Illich and others. The work of Irving Zola was particularly influential in developing the concept of medicalisation and the expansion of medicine into areas of life, including ageing, that had hitherto been considered the domain of the social and even 'natural' (Zola 1970). Consequently for Gerhardt whilst it may be true that in the early post-war years medical sociology was dominated by epidemiology, social psychology and the sociology of the medical profession, over these four phases its theoretical basis and empirical focus were transformed.

After the 1970s, in line with the greater rationalisation of health and social services, the emphasis was much more on socio-economic and political explanations of health services delivery and the organisation of healthcare institutions. Thus, medical sociology began to move away from the traditional concerns of role analysis and perspectives on human relations. There was also a greater emphasis on policy-relevant health services research and analysis of inequalities and power. However, once again older people were generally absent from these concerns. Despite this being an expansive period there were also still concerns in both the US and the UK about the discipline being an under-labourer for government and corporate medicine (Jeffreys 1991;

Bloom 2002). Today medical sociology has expanded in its aims and scope and this has led to a blossoming of academic journals, university courses, research groupings and national and international societies. Although Denny Vågero has pointed out that the discipline followed different trajectories in other European countries (Vågero 1996), the scope of medical sociology continues to expand as it addresses the rapidly changing fields of health and medicine incorporating aspects of health and development, global inequalities, transnational disease patterns and the impact of new scientific and technological developments on social relations and understandings of the body, illness and death (Shilling 1993). Perversely given its rapid development and concerns for the vulnerable and excluded and in spite of its transformed gaze, medical sociology has continued to treat old age as a separate, often peripheral category. As we shall show this lacuna is becoming increasingly difficult to maintain as the new circumstances surrounding later life start to make themselves felt not only on processes of health but on the traditional areas covered by medical sociology.

Age as a category within medical sociology

Within conventional medical sociology, when it has been addressed old age has tended to be reified as a variable (age), a period in the lifecourse (retirement), or equated with illness states (old). In spite of a continual awareness about the dangers of generalisation these conceptualisations tend to lead to later life being bracketed off as a homogenous category. This leads ultimately to static understandings of what old age and ageing represent. Examples of this can be found in two major areas of concern for medical sociologists; inequality and chronic illness.

Health inequality

With a few notable exceptions (Arber and Ginn 1993; Victor 1994; McMunn *et al*. 2006) studies of inequalities have tended to concentrate on the young (childhood) or those aged under 60. Interestingly the 'Age Stratification Model' of ageing propounded by Matilda White Riley and others in the USA during the 1970s (Riley Johnson and Foner 1972) has not generated the response that it seems it could either in America or in the UK. This is possibly because its origins were not within medical sociology or social gerontology but rather from an analytically distinct sociology of ageing. Consequently, although there is a long tradition of studying poverty in old age (Townsend 1963; Walker 1981, 2005), the extent to which health inequalities persist in later life is an area that is only now beginning to be addressed. A major part of the difficulty is that most of the research uses concepts taken from traditional health inequalities research where occupation and occupational class are taken to be important variables. This becomes more complicated in populations over retirement age where there are difficulties in measuring Socio-Economic Position (SEP) across both the lifecourse and in later life (Grundy and Holt 2001). Research now seems to suggest that inequalities in later life are beginning to converge and that this may arise as a consequence of mortality selection or survivor effects. However, the evidence is equivocal and it is difficult to untangle different effects in older populations. For example, some have argued that, after controlling for initial health status, higher levels of wealth lead to a higher probability of survival in retirement (Attanasio and Emmerson 2003). This suggests that inequalities over the lifecourse may cast a long shadow and lead to inequalities in health that persist in retirement. Analysis of the English Longitudinal Study of Ageing (ELSA) however, suggests that the length of time since labour market exit needs to be taken into account in studies of inequalities in later life (Hyde and Jones 2007). While there have always been difficulties with connecting ageing with other parts of the lifecourse it is clear to see that simple assumptions taken from theories associated with the lifecycle circumstances of older people will no longer suffice (O'Rand and Krecker 1990).

Existing studies have demonstrated a convergence in the health of those from different socio-economic positions in older age (Arber and Lahelma 1993; Arber and Ginn 1993). This is commonly explained as the result of mortality selection or survivor effects. Conversely there is other evidence to suggest that socio-economic inequalities in mortality persist into older ages (Donkin, Goldblatt and Lynch 2002) and that inequalities in morbidity continue into later life (Breeze *et al.* 2005; Grundy and Sloggett 2003). In terms of explanations for patterns of health in later life there are a number of competing hypotheses. The cumulative advantage thesis suggests that the level of health inequality related to socio-economic status in a cohort will increase as a cohort ages (Wilson, Shuey and Elder 2007). In contrast the 'divergence/convergence' hypothesis or 'age as leveller' hypothesis suggests a widening of inequalities up to early old age and a decrease in inequalities thereafter largely because of selective attrition (Beckett

2000). Although research has provided valuable insights into the relationship between lifecourse effects and health status in later life, controlling for cohort and period effects has proved problematic. This could be due to the fact that, unlike in the past, those from lower socio-economic positions are surviving into older age and, thus, carrying their increased likelihood of poorer health beyond retirement. In this sense later life, or at least the health profiles of those in later life, is coming to resemble more closely those of working age.

Furthermore, studies of the connections between lifestyle and health which have been another mainstay of health inequalities research have tended to focus on the young and middle aged, neglecting both lifestyles in later life and the inter-relationship of lifestyles choices and constraints intra- and inter-generationally. As we shall see in Chapter 2 in relation to the debates around anti-ageing techniques and the cultures of age resistance, a few notable exceptions aside (Ballard, Kuh and Wadsworth 2001), medical sociology has little to say about the subject.

Health inequalities research as a whole needs to be considered in the context of life expectancy having increased for all social classes, albeit unequally, since the 1970s. This has contributed to the formation of a more heterogeneous older population than in the past when those from lower social classes would have been at greater risk of not surviving until retirement age or dying relatively quickly afterwards. This does not preclude the possibility that socially structured differences in morbidity remain or may become more acute. The untangling of age, period and cohort effects becomes particularly difficult with respect to studies of older populations. This is because retired populations comprise cohorts that have experienced the effects of a range of political, economic and cultural events that have consequences for health status, income in retirement and levels of social participation (Evandrou and Falkingham 2000). This means that as successive cohorts enter retirement the relationship between soci-economic position (SEP) and health may change. Indeed, one of the areas medical sociology has been particularly slow to address is the relationship between length of retirement, SEP at retirement and health.

In his book *The Imprint of Time; Childhood, History and Adult Life,* Wadsworth (1991) drawing on his experience of studying birth cohorts in the UK has highlighted three aspects of time and change; the development of the individual, historical or social time passing and attachment to a particular period of time. As generations age in a rapidly changing society this may lead to changes in attitudes to and responses to patterns of health and illness. Furthermore, the social and economic determinants of (ill)health are coming under greater scrutiny as new ways of accounting for these differences are brought into play (Rose 2007a, 2007b). Those in and entering later life are not immune to these changes. In fact they play an important role in transforming our understanding of the boundaries of work, non-work, leisure and retirement that in turn have large consequences for health inequalities. Seen in this light the relative neglect of older people in health inequalities research seems odd.

Chronic illness

Sociology has made important contributions to the understanding of chronic illness based largely on research addressing the experiences and beliefs of individuals. For example, Gareth Williams (1984) opened doors for more biographical, historically engaged studies of lay understandings of chronic illness. Much of the subsequent work in this area however, has a problematic relationship with old age. Studies of chronic illness have tended to focus on disruption and disability in younger populations and biographical reconstruction is viewed in terms of normalising old age. Simon Williams' study of chronic respiratory illness (Williams 1993) while making repeated reference to the fact that the condition affects older people in different ways from younger patients does not go deeper into why this might be the case. In a similar fashion, Bury's (1982) pioneering work on biographical disruption is based on interviews with younger people who viewed arthritis as a disease of the old. This is in contrast to later work (Sanders *et al.* 2002) which, by focusing on older people with osteoarthritis, suggests that older people tend to view their disease as a 'normal' part of the lifecourse. Whilst there are many examples of research on chronic illness, the relationship between age and the experience of chronic illness remains under-theorised (Kelly and Field 1996; Williams 2000). There is however, acknowledgement of the importance of the relationship between later life and chronic conditions. Pandora Pound (Pound *et al.* 1995), in her study of older stroke survivors in working class areas of London, suggests that despite the profound physical effects of their attack informants tended to see their stroke as a normal crisis in their lives and those who had illness in the past tended to view the stroke as a form of biographical enforcement. From a life-course perspective Gareth Williams (2000) has suggested that such responses to illness in later life can be seen as a biographically anticipated event given normative expectations of ageing. We would suggest that there may also be generational effects as individuals enter later life carrying their 'generational habitus' with them (Gilleard and Higgs 2005). Socio-biographical and life history methods are used increasingly in social science to explore individual and group capacities to address social risk, to study the implications of social exclusion and consider the mobilisation of social capital (Chamberlayne, Bornat and Wengraf 2000; SOSTRIS 1999; Williams 2000, 2003). Other approaches have used modified life-grid methods to combine oral history with epidemiological background data to examine the relationship between life events and health experience (Blane 1996). In later work on quality of life in early old age (Blane, Netuveli and Bartley 2007) there is an acknowledgement of the importance of period in structuring the lives of older people. Outside of this however, there has been little work that attempts to incorporate the changes to ageing that constitute the cohort and period effects of contemporary later life. Issues such as the rise of consumerism, the importance of lifestyle and new reproductive technologies have all been addressed in reconceptualisations of medical sociology (Annandale 1998; Nettleton 2007) but the changes to ageing still seem to sit outside this gaze. Following on from this there is a need to examine the ways in which individuals in later life have become authors of their own biographies and how they construct the narrative of their lives in the context of change. As Carol Thomas (2007) reminds us, we need to be aware of the way in which sociologists interested in the study of chronic conditions have ignored alternative perspectives in favour of 'deeply rooted cultural understandings of the care and dependency needs' of 'chronically ill and disabled people' (Thomas 2007: 118). This may be as relevant for those who are older as it is for those in the disability movements.

Later life in the context of a second modernity

So far we have discussed the nature of the changes to old age and ageing but it is not sufficient to discuss these issues without looking at the structures that might lie behind them. While transformations in later life have been couched in terms of demographic transition, longevity revolution and dependency ratios, social theorists have been aware of wider secular social transformations that have been occurring over the preceding half century. This can be seen in work that addresses the changing nature of the economy, the movement from organised to disorganised capitalism (Lash and Urry 1987), the changing forms of work (Tilly and Tilly 1998; Beck 2000) and the disruptions that accompany the forces of globalisation (Held *et al.* 1999). While each approach has its own nuances, all argue that there are consequences to the decline of full employment and the disappearance of life-long careers. Institutions such as the welfare state, along with mass party politics and stable nuclear families are all thrown into flux. Social institutions, it has been argued, become more uncertain, diffuse and changeable. For example, as the sexual division of labour is questioned and becomes blurred, gender roles and the internal dynamics of families have been transformed (Beck-Gernsheim 2002; Hakim 2000; Seccombe 1993). The lifecourse has been de-institutionalised with profound consequences for retirement (Warnes 2006). Status, consumption and social security choices are increasingly de-coupled from labour force participation (Beck, Bonss and Lau 2003). Social knowledge has been restructured so that the old certainties of science, technology and rationality bump up against experiential and lay knowledge (Latour 2003). Traditional hierarchical boundaries between professionals and 'the laity' are challenged. Furthermore, the relatively separate and distinct life worlds of working class and middle class communities have been disrupted and thrown into question by new, perhaps more self-constructed, identities (Bauman 2005). Changes in social class relations and in patterns of work may be taking place against a backdrop of enduring institutions, values and cultural practices (Beynon 1999; Savage, Bagnall and Longhurst 2001). Nevertheless, these changes do present challenges to the ways in which we approach social issues. At the level of global sociology this has led to a debate concerning the development of a cosmopolitan sociology (Beck and Sznaider 2006). Crucially members of those generations entering later life today have both experienced and contributed to these social transformations. They carry their history with them into the realm of old age and in doing so transform old age itself. Such transformations however, are experienced unevenly in different parts of the world, in different localities within nation states and by different social groups.

Reflexive Modernisation or Second Modernity refers to 'the modernization of modern society' whereby older modern structures are transformed and become contingent (Beck *et al.* 2003). A number of theorists of second modernity have argued that social transformations are related to increasing individualisation coupled with a sense of self that is based on heightened knowledge about our social relations. As Bauman writes 'needing to *become* what one *is* is the feature of modern living ... Modernity replaces the *determination* of social standing with a compulsive and obligatory *self*-determination' (Bauman 2001; 144–45). From a different perspective, William Outhwaite (2006) suggests the movement towards greater individualisation and social fragmentation can be mapped on to key areas of social life. The concerns of social theory appear to be refocusing the sociological gaze away from institutions to organisations, from classes to strata and from politics to cultural issues. Theorists are less concerned with workers but with the poor/underclass, multiple and flexible identities are preferred sites of study and perhaps most controversially society as subject matter for sociological study has disappeared to be replaced with the view that society no longer exits. Whilst Outhwaite goes on to point out that there are dangers in rushing headlong into researching novel phenomena and Bryan Turner emphasises the enduring relevance of classical sociology for the understanding of social life in the twenty-first century (Turner 2006) there are still aspects of the changed circumstances of older people that have to be explained. Whilst not necessarily signing up to all aspects of the research programme of second modernity, it has many advantages at least as a starting point. For example, Beck, Bonns and Lau (2003) make explicit the importance of transnational spaces for the formation of identities. This gives rise to new tensions and conflicts. Nowhere is this more true than in the area of later life where not only is the role of the nation state in securing retirement income being challenged by globalised forms of income maintenance but also in terms of post work migration patterns. The large numbers of retired UK residents in the south of Spain is one example and the number of Canadian citizens living in Florida for part of the year is another (Katz 2005; Warnes 2006). Bauman indirectly refers to this transnational dilemma as one of being between 'tourists' and 'vagabonds' (Bauman 1998). The impact of these tensions and conflicts on the world of work has also been acutely observed by Richard Sennett (2006) and Ulrich Beck (2000), but there is little research to address the implications of these changes for retirement and later life other than suggestions that the post-war 'golden age' of state welfare is being replaced by a 'silver age' where the welfare state is much more conscious of global competitiveness, market based solutions and individual choice (Taylor-Gooby 2002). In order to make links between grand theory and empirical work Bruno Latour (Latour 2003) and Ulrich Beck (Beck, Bonss and Lau 2003) have outlined test criteria for the presence of second modernity. They suggest that there may be evidence for a multiplying of social boundaries giving rise to turbulence within and between institutions and individuals. In addition there may be an increase in the variety of claims to knowledge and forms of rationality. A focus on risk and the calculability of risk may lead to a growth in ad hoc solutions. Most importantly perhaps is Latour's postulate of the birth of the 'quasi-subject' where reflexive individuals (and these we would argue include people in later life) are expected to choose quickly from a wide range of possibilities with uncertain outcomes without the benefit of stable starting points. Whilst this may seem very radical it has the benefit of suggesting that the conditions of second modernity will be accompanied by increasing uncertainty and individualisation. This does seem to reflect some key aspects of modern times; there are more uncertain careers, less predictable lifecourses as well as new excluding practices giving rise to new forms of inequality such as that between those on private pensions and those on state pensions. In terms of social identities, individuals are called upon to become authors of their own biographies (occupational, personal and health) and construct *plausible* narratives that imbue the prevailing uncertainties with meaning and direction.

In the context of the changes to the experience of ageing outlined above, medical sociology could only benefit from considering how the experience of ageing and changes in the lifecourse might map on to such criteria. In Table 1 we summarise the test criteria for judging the impact of second modernity put forward by Beck, Latour and colleagues and relate these to research questions pertinent to the sociology of health in later life. What are the possible points of conflict in the transition to a second modernity for older people? How, for example would a more unstable lifecourse affect relationships between institutions and individuals? How would a focus on risk and side-effects affect old age and attitudes to old age? How might 'quasi-subjects' engage with growing older? What new forms of inequality might become apparent in the longevity revolution? Finally, how might biographical approaches to later life be affected by the impact of second modernity on social identities? It is not necessary to fully commit to views put forward in different ways by Latour and Beck *et al.*

to see the utility of having an over arching framework to deal with the emerging challenges of later life under new conditions. Indeed, it could be argued that other theorists such as Bauman (2000, 2005) may offer a better prism through which to describe these changes. Nevertheless it is the theorists of second modernity who are offering a research programme which brings all of these issues together.

Table 1 Criteria for understanding later life in the context of second modernity and possible research questions

Test criteria	Questions relating to later life
A multiplying of social boundaries that are purposefully created and give rise to turbulence within and between institutions and individuals.	Consider possible points of conflict and transition in the relationships between health and social care systems and older age groups. To what extent are modes of rationing and discretion being challenged and changed?
A multiplying of rationality with many different claims to knowledge.	Generations entering later life today were part of new social movements in the 1960s and 1970s. Does this give rise to more questioning of scientific approaches to ageing and later life? Do different claims to knowledge arise in the field of ageing, for example scientific, commercial and lay understandings of anti-ageing medicine?
A growth in ad hoc solutions to cope with the increasing calculation of possible side effects.	To what extent is intra- and inter-generational conflict a response to the consequences of battles over resources in late modernity?
The birth of the 'quasi-subject' where reflexive individuals are expected to choose quickly from uncertain outcomes.	Does the quasi-subject inherently reject ageing?
Increasing individualisation, uncertain careers, unstable lifecourses and new inclusive and exclusive practices creating new forms of inequality.	Is there a dark side to the culture of the third age leading to new forms of categorical inequality based on lifestyle and consumer practices?
An increasingly insecure social order where individuals become authors of their own biographies and construct fictive narratives that imbue the prevailing uncertainties with meaning.	To what extent can biographical approaches to health and illness adapt to the construction of new social identities?

Source: Adapted from Latour 2003 and Beck, Bonss and Lau 2003.

Conclusion

This chapter has identified a neglect of ageing by medical sociology both in terms of a lack of attention to the field of later life in general and through a limited construction of age and ageing as sociological categories. Addressing this neglect we would argue is not just the correcting of an oversight. It is a profound re-orientation of the sub-discipline of medical sociology. Ageing is not only becoming more salient to society and to the rest of the lifecourse but is also undergoing a process of profound change. Improvements in health and life expectancy have been accompanied by transformations in people's expectations of a post-work life that is not only viewed in terms of entitlements but also in terms of their relationship with their bodies and their identities. We will return to these themes in later chapters.

2 Social gerontology and old age

Introduction

Thomas Cole in his seminal history of ageing in America (Cole 1992) prefaces his exploration of the topic by pointing out that the current concerns for the scientific management of ageing have led to a focus on the 'problem of old age' to the detriment of other cultural dimensions of ageing. This pre-occupation with the problems of senescence is also remarked upon by Andrew Achenbaum (1995) and Stephen Katz (1996) in their accounts of the development of Gerontology as a discipline. All three writers direct attention towards ways in which both Gerontology and Geriatric Medicine have evolved to provide solutions to what has become an important dimension of social life. Katz quotes the first article in the first issue of the newly established Journal of Gerontology in 1946 which stated that 'Gerontology reflects the recognition of a new kind of problem that will increasingly command the interest and devotion of a variety of scientists, scholars, and professional workers' (Frank, 1946: 1 quoted in Katz 1996). The development of specifically social gerontological approaches to later life has followed this pattern with the US Social Science Research Council establishing a Committee on Social Adjustment in Old Age in 1944 and the Nuffield Foundation in the UK establishing a Research Unit into the Problems of Ageing at Cambridge University in 1946. These initiatives set up the trajectories for the social sciences' engagement with ageing leading to numerous surveys and research programmes including, in time, the Kansas City Study and volumes of surveys of the situation of older people in the UK. Much of the reason for this problem-associated approach lies not in the vicissitudes of old age, for which there had been much policy and action over previous centuries, but in the emergence of a distinct part of the lifecourse called retirement particularly in the USA in the 1940s (Graebner 1980) and the 1960s in the UK (Harper and Thane 1989). This development led some sociologists such as Parsons (1942) and Burgess (1960) to worry about the 'roleless role' of the retired person which had come into being as a result of the self-regulating functional specialisation of modern societies. Although such an approach to later life may owe more to 'functionalist' theoretical assumptions about the nature of the relationship between roles, social functions and the reproduction of social structures, it is nevertheless true that mass consumer societies such as post-war America had indeed created a population defined not so much through their indigence but by their exit from the labour market. Obviously this state referred mainly to men for whom social role and employment were seen as largely interchangeable whereas a consistent domesticated role was assumed for women. However, the circumstances surrounding retired people were not such that they could be left to be permanently in a state of limbo. Into this breach stepped an approach which, while still focusing on the social adjustment of the older person, saw many of the same features through the prism of 'disengagement' theory (Cumming and Henry 1961). Theorising the wider processes that went alongside retirement, it hypothesised that older people in industrial societies disengaged themselves from the roles that they occupied in order that younger generations would have similar opportunities to develop and take on their socially necessary roles. Consequently disengagement was assumed to not only occur in relation to work roles but also in relation to families, when retired generations became much less central to the lives of their children. Focusing on a psychological approach, disengagement theory saw itself as influenced by the work of Erik Erikson and notions of life review (Erikson 1959). It was assumed that disengagement was a universal process defined by the interconnectedness between later life and death. A considerable amount of research was undertaken in the USA during the 1960s to provide evidence for this theory. A longitudinal study in Kansas City (Neugarten *et al.* 1964) showed that older people did indeed disengage, although women started this process at widowhood whereas men began on retirement. Again, the processes were seen as involving difficulties in the *roles* being played by older people and the answers in psychological adaptation. This approach, which for a long time was one of the dominant paradigms in social gerontology, saw the way in which old age occurred in modern societies as an inevitable and natural process. Questions about whether older people wanted to 'disengage' or were forced to do so by society were not asked. The emphasis on psychological adjustment also avoided looking at the very real social processes that structured old age. Moreover, as time went on, many of the researchers involved in studying the phenomena including Bernice Neugarten (1996) began to conclude that many of the assumptions of disengagement theory were wrong in both interpretation and inference. Others concluded that the ideas were over generalised, did not describe a unitary phenomenon and avoided dealing with issues of power (Hochschild 1975).

Structured dependency theory

If the disengagement approach centred on the perspective of the individual older person, then the analysis put forward by the predominantly British 'structured dependency' school (Townsend 1981) stressed the importance of social policy. Here the problem of old age was not one of social adjustment but of a 'structured' dependency. For writers in this school and those who described themselves as adopting the 'political economy' approach to ageing (Walker 1981; Phillipson 1982; Estes 1979) the circumstances of retirement were the ones that most defined the older person and were ones set by government social policy. The age of entitlement to a state retirement pension marked the onset of old age at both individual and social levels. The arbitrariness of the age at which this occurs is demonstrated by its variability in different countries and the fact that it is currently set to progressively move up in the UK over the next few decades.

Townsend noted that not only does retirement mark a withdrawal from the formal labour market but it also marks a shift from making a living through earning a wage to being someone dependent on a replacement income. That this income was often funded by the State demonstrated the role of social policy in structuring the dependency that many older people fell into. In the UK the relatively low levels at which the state pension was paid out at indicated the low priority older people had in decisions about state welfare. But as Alan Walker (1981) and others pointed out, the continuing impact of social class into later life was also indicated in the relative imbalance between the level of state retirement pensions which funded the majority of working class retirees' old age and the amounts paid out by the better-funded occupational pensions enjoyed by the middle class. Old age was seen as an extension of employment policy and framed around the need to prevent an overlap between pensioners and workers. This is evident in the fact that in the UK until the 1990s it was a requirement that to receive a State retirement pension the recipient could not undertake paid employment without running the risk that the money be deducted from his or her pension (Hill 2007). Pensioners consequently were equated with the unemployed and seen as a residual category of the population drawing resources from public funds. Focusing on policy led to considerable interest in researching poverty in later life. In many respects this continued earlier traditions of social surveys carried out by Rowntree in the first half of the twentieth century (Rowntree 1901, 1947). However, while these earlier reports were designed to alert the public to the circumstances experienced by older people in Britain, much of the research on poverty in later life that took place in the 1950s and beyond was more interested in pointing out how one of the key aspirations of the Welfare State was not being met. The persistence of poverty in later life belied the idea of 'cradle to the grave' social security and seriously undermined the promise of social citizenship. For most of the 1950s, 1960s and 1970s, governments in the UK did not seriously improve the level of the state retirement pension or address the poverty that accompanied it – a situation made worse during the period of high inflation that was part of the economic recession of the 1970s. In these conditions the circumstances faced by pensioners were very much the direct outcome of government social policies. The failure by successive administrations to uprate pension benefits in line with rises in average earnings was another example of the structuring of dependency in old age. Evandrou and Falkingham (1993) calculated that by the mid-nineties the state retirement pension was only worth 20 per cent of average earnings and that this would decline to less than 10 per cent by 2020.

Structured dependency is not just limited to the economic sphere but also pervades social processes as an effect of the inferior status accorded to older people. Taking the core ideas further Townsend (1986) argued that the association of age with infirmity and dependency not only 'represents' the position of older people but also justifies the exclusion of older people from various forms of social participation. Ageism also emerges out of the cultural valorisation of 'youthfulness' which not only defines ageing in negative terms but also clears the way to make it acceptable to discriminate against older people. This can manifest itself in policies seeking to limit medical or healthcare resources to older people, in discriminatory employment practices and in the treatment of physically frail or mentally confused older people (Townsend 1986).

For writers such as Townsend and Walker the 'disengaged' position of later life is not only a social construction but also something that should be challenged by campaigns for the restoration of full citizenship rights to older people and by the re-invigoration of a much better funded State Retirement Pension (Townsend and Walker 1995). This position has been seen as increasingly anachronistic given that the general move in government policy has been towards downplaying the State Retirement Pension in securing later life and emphasising individual responsibility for achieving a comfortable post-retirement income. However, structured dependency theory still pitches itself as being committed to the pursuit of a more egalitarian approach to later life and sees, in this increasingly individualised approach to pensions, forces that perpetuate class and gender inequalities. Taking class inequality as their cue, the 'political economy' strand has linked the position of older people to more neo-Marxist themes around the role of older person within the capitalist economy (Phillipson 1982; Walker 1981). Equally gender inequality in relation to pensions has been explored (Ginn and Arber 2001). In more recent works the mixed fortunes of older people in the globalised economy have been a focus for theorising (Estes, Biggs and Phillipson 2003). However, Walker in his reconsideration of his earlier work (Walker 2005) runs the risk of extending the political economy approach to the point where it becomes so generalised that it loses its explanatory power or indeed its critical insight.

The third age

The problematising of old age does not just have to be around perceived role deficits or social exclusion; it can also be about the responsibilities that older generations should take on as they enjoy a fulfilling 'third age' of relative good health and affluence. The idea of the third age is most associated with the work of Peter Laslett (1989 republished in 1996 in a revised format) who argued in his *A Fresh Map of Life* that later life can no longer be viewed in the pessimistic fashion that has previously been the case. Not only is the portion of most people's lives spent in retirement increasing, but the idea of a fixed retirement age has been challenged by the many individuals who have chosen to take retirement at ages other than that set by the State for Retirement Pension eligibility. For many, Laslett argued, retirement offers possibilities for undertaking the self-enriching activities denied earlier in life when the tasks of earning a living or bringing up children, or both, got in the way.

> The life phase in which there is no longer employment and child raising to commandeer time, and before morbidity enters to limit activity and mortality brings everything to a close, has been called the Third Age. Those in this phase have passed through a first age of youth, when they are prepared for the activities of maturity, and a second age of maturity, when their lives were given to those activities, and have reached a third age in which they can, within fairly wide limits, live their lives as they please, before being overtaken by a fourth age of decline.
>
> (Laslett 1996: 3)

This division of the lifecourse into a succession of ages is not necessarily new or indeed easy to operationalise – a fact that Laslett acknowledged. In positing a long positive third age underpinned by relative good health and a short but ultimately terminal fourth age there is an opening up of the period of retirement away from the simple conflation of retirement and old age. As we go on to discuss in later chapters this notion of the fourth age as defining an old age of decrepitude and decline may be intrinsically connected to the existence of a third age but it is analytically separate. Laslett refers to the fourth age but does not wish to dwell on it other than to wish that it be a short terminal period. However, in focusing on the third age Laslett is wary that later life should not become self-indulgent. To this end there are warnings regarding the dangers of indolence and the importance of accepting the responsibilities of the third age.

> Let us look once again at the characters of those responsibilities ... First and foremost, it must be said that the British elderly have an overwhelming responsibility to persuade, to cajole, to insist that their country and its population learn to be their age. It is a responsibility clearly shared with all other citizens, but rests particularly upon them. Their further obligation, however, is entirely personal. It is to fulfill themselves as far as

personal circumstances and history permits, to use their Third Age in fact in ways which have been suggested here.

(Laslett 1989: 197)

In particular, Laslett identifies education as one of the key areas necessary for a successful third age and to this end he was a proponent of the University of the Third Age and saw that its activities were very much the spirit of the third age. He also saw the duties of the third age as going much further than just using time well and explicitly called for older people to act as cultural trustees for society in general and for the preservation of craft skills in particular (Laslett 1989: 196–203). The challenge, as Laslett sees it, is to get those in the third age to accept their responsibilities rather than simply enjoy a leisure retirement.

This moral reading of the third age has become more difficult to maintain as a conflation between the third age and the baby boomers has become widely accepted, particularly in the US (Freedman 1999; Gilleard and Higgs 2007b). This conflation transforms retirement into an arena of lifestyle and consumption rather than education and responsibility. A blurring of the distinction between 'middle' and 'old' age is fostered by the increasing influence of lifestyle consumerism on significant numbers of people outside of the younger age groups typically associated with these developments (Featherstone and Hepworth 1991). Instead of a desire to use the advantages of the third age for the benefit of society, it is seen as a way to avoid old age itself and extending an ill-defined middle age further and further along the lifecourse. The submergence of clear age-appropriate divisions in dress, along with the greater acceptability of leisure clothing has meant that jeans and t-shirts can be worn by people of very different ages without social sanction (Twigg 2007). Featherstone and Hepworth (1991) advance the idea that these processes are related to individuals negotiating the changing circumstances of later life where signs of old age become seen as a 'mask' detracting from the person beneath. While we will deal with these issues later in this book, at this point it is sufficient to point out that Laslett sets up the third age in terms that are as much about the moral duties of older people as they are about new opportunities.

Productive ageing

The implicit concerns regarding the status of older people under the changed circumstances of contemporary retirement has also been a theme of what has come to be known as the 'productive aging' approach (Hinterlong, Morrow-Howell and Sherraden 2001). This position has antecedents specifically in Rowe and Kahn's notion of 'successful aging' (1987, 1998) which sought to separate this positive state from what was termed 'usual' ageing. Inspiring a whole series of studies within the clinical and social sciences searching for markers of success in ageing, 'successful aging' has been criticised for an overtly individualistic approach to what counts as success and failure (Cruikshank 2003).

Taking a broader approach, productive ageing was concerned with the fact that not only were larger numbers of people living longer and healthier lives but that changes in the nature of work, particularly in relation to information and communications technologies (ICT), were making it possible for older people to make significant social or economic contributions rather than retiring to a state of total leisure. Again the focus was on social engagement with the idea of productive ageing extended to go beyond conventional meanings of productivity including volunteering and civic participation (Burr, Caro and Moorhead 2001). Older people acting in this way would therefore demonstrate that they were not just consumers of resources but also made a valuable contribution to the societies in which they lived. The benefits of engaging in productive ageing for the individual were considerable as they not only engaged individuals in society but also utilised otherwise underused capacities and capabilities. Obviously proponents of the approach were aware that there needed to be caution regarding the limits to such productive ageing and that older people were not obliged or exploited in undertaking activities. Many of the criticisms of the productive ageing approach did indeed focus on this aspect pointing out that the laudable intentions could easily be interpreted as a simple invocation of the need to be productive in conventional economic terms (Holstein 1999). Estes and Mahakian (2001) go further in their criticism by linking both successful and productive ageing approaches to an extension of market principles into the process of ageing itself which act to benefit what they call the 'bio-medically orientated medical-industrial complex' and ignore the social and economic disadvantages operating in both society and social policy (Estes and Mahakian 2001: 210). As a result, while the advocates of the productive ageing approach have moved the debate on ageing away from a simple equation of age and dependency, there is still a tendency to identify those aspects of later life that mesh with normative assumptions about social and economic worth as desirable.

Equally there is, accordingly, a tendency to downplay the contradictions implicit in this trajectory most notably among those who cannot or do not want to play this role or who are already socially disadvantaged.

Cultures of ageing

Not all approaches to the questions of contemporary old age project later life as a problem to be solved. Gilleard and Higgs (2000) have argued that a 'cultures of ageing' approach based on the increasing cultural engagement with lifestyle and consumerism by successive cohorts of retirees would fit better with the new realities of ageing. This suggests that we are witnessing the ageing of generations who have taken a particular approach to adult life which has been organised through the prism of a youth-orientated consumer culture. The post-war 'baby bulge' cohorts who grew up in circumstances of expanding consumer choice and economic prosperity created a 'generational schism' between themselves and those older than them who had grown up in less prosperous times. This schism manifested itself in attitudes, music and clothes but most significantly in lifestyles where there have been cumulative changes to the nature of families, relationships and sexuality. An important part of this 'generational habitus' (Gilleard and Higgs 2005) is that it has not been discarded as the teenagers of the sixties became the retirees of the twenty-first century. It is this generationally located set of dispositions that Gilleard and Higgs see as being behind many of the features of contemporary ageing. The identification of retirement in terms of its opportunities for leisure rather than simply being a 'roleless role' or a moment for life review can be seen by the fact that a significant proportion of older workers do not wait until the State Retirement Pension age to retire. Retirement as choice is valorised by this culture while those who face redundancy or conventional retirement patterns are seen as less agentic and less able to deal with the new circumstances of later life. While conventional retirement and later life still continues, for many they exist in the shadow of a hegemonic concept of a third age which establishes the expectations and values for post-work life. That contemporary retirement is influenced by these cultural pressures can be seen in the worries of governments and social commentators as they seek to reflect this image of later life. Indeed it is the emphasis on leisure retirement over civic participation as a key motivation in later life that prompted Laslett to worry about the capacity of the Third Age to maintain its moral underpinning. Similar concerns can be seen in the writings of those advocating productive ageing. Will the 'greedy geezers' take the resources without reciprocating is a question that motivates much of the research agenda (Butler 2002). In addition, later life is increasingly bound up with a self-perpetuating concept of youth culture which is now engaging with old age itself. It is not just the individualised 'mask' of ageing that needs to be understood but the whole generationally saturated social terrain on which ageing occurs. Gilleard and Higgs make a point of arguing that the issues of individual ageing are at the centre of a number of cultural processes regarding the undesirability of being identified as 'old' or being seen in terms of a category of 'lack'. This not only leads to growing opportunities for the development of an anti-ageing industry and its products but also leads to a greater emphasis on the plasticity of the body. Themes, products and techniques which increasingly reach back across the age spectrum ensure that the impact of cultures of ageing is felt at earlier and earlier ages.

While an emphasis on the physical signs of the ageing body is an important aspect of the social changes accompanying the reconstitution of old age, such concerns are only one dimension of it. Echoing themes from the third age and productive ageing, it is also equally important that no activities are seen to exist outside the ambition or capabilities of older people, whether it is running a marathon or as the 77-year-old former astronaut John Glenn has done, going back into space or having children post-menopausally. The removal of ideas of age-inappropriate activities or clothing illustrates the connections between third-age lifestyles, consumerism and consumer culture. As the cultural distinctions previously dominated by social class are replaced by individually focused lifestyles, the consequences of ageing become one of the principal arenas where identity is played out.

Gilleard and Higgs (2000) have been criticised for overplaying agency and underplaying structure in their descriptions of later life (Walker 2005). In particular the transformation of later life along the lines that they describe depends on older people having the resources to be able to participate in the various cultural activities now open to them. While the incomes and standard of living of the majority of retired people in the EU and North America have improved greatly over the past few decades this affluence has not necessarily been equally shared. However, this does not mean that these cultural processes are not happening or do not impact on the majority of people in later life. Rather ignoring these changes means that older people are once again identified as a category of social policy needing intervention rather than accepting that there is now a diversity of locations within the older population, some of whom are not as well off as others. This criticism does illuminate the difficulties that arise as a consequence of old age being an unstable phenomenon which is constantly changing. The dispositions of current retirees cannot be assumed to continue indefinitely as some of the unique factors associated with the 'baby bulge' generation may disappear. However, it is also difficult to imagine that later life will return to the circumstances that marked out the problem of 'old age' in the early decades of the twentieth century. There will be different ways of seeing the problems of 'old age' in the future but it is possibly more fruitful to see ageing as having moved from the margins of society to occupying a central position and that ageing will be seen as the multi-faceted topic that it is.

Social research and the problematisation of later life

The perception of older people as a social problem has a long history in both social and health research, leading to a perception that having an older population can only be a disaster for the nation that finds itself in this unfortunate position. In the immediate post-war period Alfred Sauvy suggested that Britain's economic difficulties were largely the result of an ageing population. Furthermore he went on:

> The danger of a collapse of western civilization owing to a lack of replacement of its human stock cannot be questioned. Perhaps we ought to regard this organic disease, this lack of vitality of the cells, as a symptom of senility of the body politic itself and thus compare social biology with animal biology.
>
> (Sauvy 1947: 124)

This sense of foreboding had been a strong theme driving earlier developments in social policy. The introduction of old age pensions in Britain in 1908 was not only intended to eliminate extreme poverty in old age but also to lower 'poor law' expenditure on older people (McNicol and Blaikie 1989). If social research during the nineteenth and early twentieth century had established that old age represented a problem it was further complicated by the difficulty of separating out the elderly from paupers. In other words distinguishing the deserving and 'thrifty' from those whose circumstances were of their own making was one of the main tasks of the means test. While this entitlement problem had been at the heart of much Victorian social policy and continued all through the inter-war period, by the mid-1920s the effects of the economic depression had moved the terms of debate in the direction of the capacity of retirement to alleviate unemployment. In this formulation removal from active participation in the workforce was the main motivation for retirement and led in time to a lowering of the retirement age to 65.

In the USA, the drivers for change were similar in their concern to take older workers out of the workforce, however the fact that the majority of older people were in employment complicated matters. The Depression of the 1930s created an impetus for change but not only had legislators to deal with the added complication of the federal structure of the nation, but also with the confusing pattern of Civil War pension entitlements that many different people were eligible for. On top of this many companies and occupations operated a whole array of different pension schemes (Achenbaum 1978; Graebner 1980). It was not even the case that there was one dominant approach to the funding of later life. The Townsendite movement of the 1930s, named after Dr Francis E. Townsend, argued for a tax-funded state pension rather than one based on a contributory principle. Furthermore, in advocating the reflationary potential of creating a large number of state-funded consumers it reconceptualised retirement with the slogan '*youth for work / age for leisure*' (Graebner 1980: 194). The New Deal and its Social Security pension when it was established in 1935 was much more conventional in its conception acting as both a poverty alleviation programme and as a way of dealing with unemployment by releasing employment to younger workers.

The identification of the old as a problem to be resolved continued in this light for much of the second half of the twentieth century although with different national emphases. In the UK the tradition that includes Rowntree's studies of poverty (1901, 1947) continued in the work of Townsend (1963) and has been a continuing theme of social gerontologists into the twenty-first century (Bardasi, Jenkins and Rigg 2002). Conversely in the USA the successful selling of retirement after the Second World War led, as we have seen, to a whole series of research initiatives and programmes on both successful and productive ageing, investigating adaptation to the circumstances of retirement. Whatever the national differences, the collection of data to answer questions posed as the 'problem of ageing' has continued apace albeit now within the context of population ageing and the economic consequences that accompany it. Paradoxically this has meant that research is now directed at the problems posed by 'a rapidly growing population of rather healthy and self-sufficient persons whose collective dependence is now straining the economies of western nations' (Katz 1996: 128).

Bio-gerontological perspectives

This agenda has been more pronounced among the biomedical and applied research communities as it has entailed a shift from a focus on poverty towards discussions of what can be expected of ageing bodies and whether or not the past is a good basis for predictions of the future. Again there are echoes of the debates surrounding structured dependency and productive ageing with pessimistic views about the burden of ageing populations being replaced by concerns as to whether the health of today's older population is time limited or can be sustained and the degree to which individuals must become the agents of their own health in later life. From the bio-gerontological point of view, there are many like Tom Kirkwood (1999) who argue that the human lifespan is malleable, mortality only occurring as a result of an accumulation of damage in cells and tissues and limitations in investments in somatic maintenance. More controversially writers such as Aubrey de Grey argue that longevity can be extended upwards once the basic biological processes have been understood (de Grey 2007). Based on ideas of what he terms 'engineered negligible senescence' which aims to overcome what he sees as the seven causes of ageing, which range from cancer to cell loss, his views have been heavily criticised but not necessarily refuted. While these views may still be at the outer limits of bio-gerontology, at a population level there is now a widespread recognition that rates of death as a consequence of infectious disease have been dropping in the most prosperous nations since the early part of the twentieth century and that chronic illness rates especially among the older population have replaced them as a healthcare concern (Omran 2005). That increased longevity might lead to higher rates of morbidity and/or disability has been seen as a product of the 'failure of success' where industrial societies have passed through an epidemiological transition which has shifted the burden of disease onto chronic conditions in later life

(Crimmins 2004). However, while this conclusion might fit in well with Jonathan Swift's view of the immortal Struldbrugs who may have had eternal life but not eternal youth thus being condemned to a life of unmitigated misery, it has been challenged by evidence that does not suggest that increased life expectancy comes at the cost of an 'expansion of morbidity' (Fogel 1994). Writers such as James Fries have proposed a thesis built around a 'compression of morbidity' where even under the conditions of increased life expectancy the proportion of life spent in ill health is concentrated into an ever shorter period prior to death (Fries 1980; Fries 2003). While this view challenged many of the assumptions made about the connection between ageing and chronic illness there has been considerable support for the claim that chronological age in itself is not a factor in increasing levels of disability and chronic illness (Manton and Gu 2001). Although analysis based on *subjective* measures of health has suggested an increasing disease burden in later life (ONS 2004) more objective indicators of disability suggest a more positive view of healthy life expectancy (Schoeni, Freedman and Martin 2008). Nevertheless, discussion about future pressures on healthcare use has generated the most concern. People aged 65 and over account for just under half of total hospital and community health spending in England (Evandrou 2005) and the Wanless report on healthcare demand in the UK estimated that there would be a 57 per cent rise in the number of dependent older people during 2001–31 (Wanless 2001). The report's authors argue that, based on these figures, places in residential care will need to expand from around 400,000 in 1996 to 450,000 by 2010 and 670,000 by 2031. Consequently, the Wanless Report while being aware that there is evidence for the compression of morbidity in the UK population and that most healthcare costs are incurred in an individual's last year of life, still concludes that an ageing population is going to put increasing strains on publicly funded healthcare. To this must be added the emergence of an 'obesity epidemic' which may reverse the upward trend in both mortality and disability and may lead to new patterns of chronic illness. Olshansky *et al.* (2005) argue that current trends in obesity in the US may result in a decline in life expectancy for future cohorts. Based on current rates of death associated with obesity they predict that life expectancy will be reduced by between one-third and three-quarters of a year. Concerns over diet and exercise reflect an increasing emphasis on individualised accounts of health behaviour. This has led Blaxter (2000) to argue that trends toward individualisation in the later half of the twentieth century led to people constructing their lives in terms of ahistorical private health trajectories. Health lifestyles have been defined as 'collective patterns of health related behaviour based on choices from options available to people according to their life chances' (Cockerham, Rütten and Abel 1997: 321). There is a growing body of evidence suggesting that class related lifestyles have a long-term effect on the patterning of illness and mortality and this is related to age, period and cohort effects. For example, in the UK, increases in liver cirrhosis mortality rates over the last 50 years have been linked to changes in alcohol consumption over the same period (Leon and McCambridge 2006). While life expectancy improved rapidly over the last 30 years, class differences in mortality from lifestyle related diseases persist. A prospective study of men aged between 65 and 85 years at follow up found that absolute differences in mortality between social class groups fell in the last quarter of the twentieth century but that relative differences may have increased over the same period (Ramsay *et al.* 2008). The trends are complex. In Canada a study of health lifestyles among baby boomers identified a number of contradictory trends. A substantial fall in smoking rates, excessive drinking and lack of exercise over the last quarter of the twentieth century was accompanied by a sharp increase in rates of obesity and diabetes (Wister 2005). Manton (1982) uses the notion of 'dynamic equilibrium' to suggest that mortality in later life is affected by the rate of 'natural ageing' and the distribution of risk factors for specific diseases in the population. Interventions aimed at risk factors will bring improvements in both mortality and reduce the severity of associated disabilities. Schoeni, Freedman and Martin (2008) have noted how changes in smoking behaviour, greater educational attainment and declines in poverty have affected the decline in disability levels in the USA. This however again prompts recourse to discourses regarding the achievement of a successful later life as the province of the fortuitous (cumulatively advantaged) and the disciplined rather than the expectation of the ordinary person.

Following on from this there has been a continuing gerontological research interest in charting the levels of individual functioning and decline among those coming under the gaze of appropriate health and social services. As Victor (2006) points out, the pattern of morbidity can differ from the pattern of mortality leading to very different categories of health problems particularly where high morbidity is connected to low mortality such as with musculoskeletal disease and dementia. This has led to a concern with the interpretation and measurement of Quality of Life (QoL) particularly among the most vulnerable groups of older people. One difficulty has always been the separation of QoL from the influences upon it, particularly when they are related to health (Higgs *et al.* 2003). It is not surprising then that while much research is directed at finding the positive aspects of the lives of particular groups of older people, there is a constant backdrop that individuals are adapting to negative circumstances in their assessment of QoL. This may often be the case but once again the older person's position is problematised in relation to the population as a whole and the gerontologist's role is to bring this aspect of social life to the attention of society or at least to professionals and policy makers.

Another factor may in fact be institutional. In the UK the specialty of geriatric medicine has dominated the field of the healthcare of older people. Owing much to the specific organisational features of British healthcare, not least the establishment of the National Health Service after the Second World War, geriatric medicine was slowly established through battles over territory and disciplinary boundaries from the 1930s onwards (Evans 1997; Barton and Mulley 2003). From a small base it grew to be one of the largest specialties in the NHS in terms of the number of consultants employed and the number of training places offered. At the same time, old age psychiatry developed from the 1940s onwards marking a shift away from neuro-pathology in older mental hospital inmates to address need and to oversee care in the community (Hilton 2005). In both specialties there was a direct link to the pre-NHS poor law healthcare institutions through the large numbers of long-stay beds that these specialties inherited. While this situation has in the most part been transformed with both beds and responsibilities diminishing with the changes to the older population, it may be that the priorities established through a focus on the needs of the chronically sick have left their mark on social gerontology.

Conclusion

In this chapter we have attempted to delineate the tendency within Gerontology to problematise the circumstances of later life either through theoretical accounts of adjustment, disengagement, dependency or poverty. Equally life expectancy, mortality, morbidity and disability rates are conceptualised in terms of the potential difficulties that are brought about as the population ages. As later life becomes more of a positive experience for greater numbers of people such a problematising approach is not the most useful prism for viewing contemporary later life. We suggest that the changing relations of ageing need to be seen both in terms of changes to mortality, morbidity and the health of older people as well as the generational habitus of the cohorts now entering retirement. These 'new' older people challenge much of the thinking about later life and how it relates to gerontology as well as to the study of health and the somatic society.

3   The body at later ages

Introduction

The association between the physical appearance of the ageing body and notions of tragedy can be traced back to ancient Greece (Fox 2006) suggesting that negative attitudes to bodily ageing are not just a consequence of the youth-based obsessions of modern societies. However, as Turner (1991) has argued, time and memory are more problematic in modern societies and in a period of rapid social change our cultural references are rapidly transformed into the stuff of nostalgia so that, in his words, to become old is to be 'museumized' (Turner 1991: 253). For Turner this is strongly related to the *pace* of generational change. Consequently, individual experiences of, as well as meanings attached to, ageing bodies need to be understood in the social context of generational habitus. As we have argued in Chapter 1, second modernity refers to a radicalisation of modernity itself; a dominant feature of which is an increasing emphasis on individualisation and self-regulation, as well as self-discipline and the purposeful and continuous re-working of individual identities (Bauman 2000; Beck, Giddens and Lash 1994; Beck 2006). This is closely related to the rise of the 'will to health' and the 'somatisation of the self' where the body, body maintenance and body image are at the centre of social relations (Rose 2001). The body emerges as a site for regulatory work but, according to Turner, instead of traditional religious-based discipline, within a secular consumer culture, the body is treated as a site of surface impressions and ultimately becomes a sacred concern. In this context the aged body is interpreted as a sign of failure and, as Sennett (2006) argues, old age brings with it the spectre of uselessness. There are contradictions here of course in that a culture of ageing also opens up possibilities for new lifestyles, activities and meanings while at the same time closing down opportunities (Gilleard and Higgs 2000, 2005).

This chapter considers attempts within the sociology of health and illness to address the body or bodies at later ages. Since Shilling (1993) referred to the body as an absent presence within sociology, considerable theoretical and empirical work has been undertaken to try to address this lacuna; but until recently very little of this work addressed ageing bodies (Twigg 2004). In fact, both ageing and the body have been neglected fields within sociology and before Shilling made his prescient remark Turner (1991) had already argued that the absence of ageing in sociology could be attributed to the absence of a sociology of the body (p. 245). While work that draws on the traditions of medical sociology has focused on the problem of embodiment (Williams 2003) much of the recent literature on ageing has focused on social attitudes to the appearance of old age within postmodern culture (Gullette 2004; Woodward 1991). Such work has challenged 'taken for granted' understandings of ageing but does not fully engage with the ageing body. In this chapter therefore we review work on the sociology of the body and draw on critical realist theory to develop a critique of postmodern accounts of ageing bodies. Following this we turn to work that attempts to situate sociological accounts of the body in the context of second modernity and consider the implications of the rise of the reflexive self and the vicissitudes of ageing bodies for the lived experience of disability.

Sociology of the body and embodiment

Within the Sociology of Health and Illness, researching and theorising the body has received an impetus from two key developments. First, there is the impact of advances in medical science and new medical technologies (NMTs) which have led to novel challenges to understandings of the body and of bodily boundaries. Second, as previously mentioned, a secular transformation of social structures has led to an increasing emphasis on the body as a source of identity and as a site for self-regulation. It is increasingly recognised that our social experiences and social environment can have profound effects upon our bodies and our bodies in turn impact upon the social. Contrary to the accounts of popular science, our bodies are not simply biological mechanisms that are separate from social context; rather they are engaged in the continuous reproduction of the social (Rose and Rose 2001; Higgs and Jones 2003). Social theorists have grappled with the problem of the inter-relationship between a material body and individual subjectivity from a variety of perspectives (Annandale 1998). Rejecting the mind–body dualism of Cartesian thought, many commentators have adopted the concept of embodiment as a means of explaining the dialectical relationship between the body and individual perception. Following Merleau-Ponty (2002 [1962]) it can be argued that embodiment refers to the lived experience of both having a body and being a body and describes the 'bodily bases' of the action and interaction of individuals and groups. Turner (1991, 1996) for example, has argued that the centrality of our bodies to our experience was at the core of Merleau-Ponty's phenomenology and he drew on his work to suggest that in being 'open to the world' we subjectively hold on to our youthful bodily self-image and consequently lack empathy with older people, or at least people who look old, even when we ourselves are old. With respect to embodiment and later life, research with ballet dancers has informed the view that the body is at the core of the ontology of ageing, placing increasing limits on individual agency as we age (Wainwright and Turner 2006). While such research has produced useful insights, it may be overly focused on the performative aspects of body-work and in particular provides romanticised and valorised accounts of individual responses to pain and decline. Other work on embodiment and ageing has focused on the experiences of athletes and used Bourdieu's work to postulate the concept of an 'age Habitus' (Tulle 2007). Formulated in this fashion, however, age habitus seems to contradict Bourdieu's own conceptualisation in that it locates 'habitus' at a certain point in the lifecycle rather than being structured and structuring across the lifecycle. Again, while offering useful theoretical insights, there is a danger here of generalising from the specific and ignoring the social context, for example, the ways in which an activity such as long-distance running promotes forms of embodiment that legitimise class relations and 'naturalises' inequalities, be they based on age, gender or social background (Abbas 2004).

Much work on the sociology of the body emphasises the importance of body image for social interactions. In Goffman's work, for example, the body is conceived as the basis for the presentation of the self in the social world (Goffman 1969). The body is seen as a material entity which individuals are able to control and call upon as a resource to facilitate social interaction. He argued that the meanings attached to the body are determined by shared understandings of body idiom. Here, body idiom refers to non-verbal communications that form a basis for social conventions and includes what we wear, deportment, physical gestures and emotional expression. These shared vocabularies enable us to make sense of the way in which someone presents his or herself and are often used as a basis for categorising individuals. These ideas have much in common with Bourdieu's work on bodily practices as a source and site of social distinction (Bourdieu 1984). But, for Goffman, the body acts as a means of mediating the relationship between people's self-identity and their social identity, in other words mediating between personality and social status. This link between the body and identity has been picked up in the work of Shilling (1993) who argues that 'The social meanings which are attached to particular bodily forms and performances tend to become internalized and exert a powerful influence on an individual's sense of self and feelings of inner worth' (Shilling 1993: 83).

Research on the way the ageing body is portrayed and understood is limited, but work by Bytheway and Johnson (1998) on images from cartoons, photographs, magazines and advertisements has highlighted the manner in which the realities of ageing are distorted through Bourdieu's concept of symbolic violence where representations are imbued with considerable power. However, representations of the body and body image are also fluid and dynamic phenomena that change over the lifecourse. With respect to ageing bodies, Featherstone (1991) suggested that there were two underlying themes to the cultural representation of ageing. The first he referred to as 'heroic' youthful body maintenance which is a feature of consumer society. He made strong links between these cultural representations and consumer-based concerns with longevity, rejuvenation and activities aimed at refurbishing the outer surface of the body. For those who are unable to meet the high standards of this consumerist imperative, whose bodies fail them as they grow older and who become trapped in decrepitude; the second connected theme applies and the body becomes a prison. Featherstone uses the metaphor of the 'mask of ageing' to suggest the ways in which individuals are constrained by their outward appearance. The outward appearance of the body has also been a focus of much writing for those working within the social constructionist tradition with post-structuralist writers in particular viewing the body as the textual outcome of discourses (Grosz 1994, 1995). Here much is made of discourses that set up binary differentiations between bodies such as fat/thin, male/female, young/old and the powerful discourse of bio-medicine is particularly criticised for its role in defining healthy and unhealthy bodies through discourses of scientific normality/abnormality. The echoes of the work of Michel Foucault are ever present. In the hands of Foucault, the body is constructed through discourses of power and becomes a site for surveillance with medicine being viewed as having a moral and epistemological as well as a clinical purpose. Individual bodies are trained and observed and populations are monitored through the activities of social institutions such as prisons, hospitals, schools and clinics that continually produce and monitor knowledge of bodies. Through the clinical gaze bodies are objectified and assessed according to standards of the 'normal' and this knowledge informs social policies which, in turn, are directed towards controlling bodies. This perspective has been extended by Armstrong (1995) who suggested that while the clinical gaze in the late nineteenth and early twentieth century delved deeper within individual bodies, in the late twentieth century the gaze also extended outwards to the body politic covering the surveillance of whole populations. In the twenty-first century the gaze may change again as advances in pharmacogenetics offer up opportunities for drugs to be tailored to individual genetic profiles. These insights are taken further by Turner (1996) who unpicks the different ways in which the body is produced and regulated in society. The body becomes a central field of political and cultural activity. Policies of neo-liberal states become oriented towards governmentality, or the 'conduct of conduct', and the social order is increasingly built around behavioural control, regulation of bodies, internal restraint of desire and physical presentation and representation (Dean 1999). In this way bodies are regulated by means of a range of available technologies, by individuals as well as agents of the state, in order to meet the needs of rationalised capitalism.

In the context of a society whose focus is on monitoring health and valorising an outwardly healthy appearance, illness makes the body problematic. Illness sets limits to social action and has a profound impact on identity and identity (re)construction. The bodily effects of illness and impairment and the consequences for the self have been considered in relation to illness narratives and styles of adjustment (Bury 1982); death and dying (Elias 1985); the emotions (Williams and Bendelow 1998); and the gendered nature of meanings attached to bodies, including attitudes to ageing bodies and the gendered division of labour within body work and personal care (Twigg 2002). Illness also raises issues of bodily boundaries and the ways in which notions of dirt and hygiene are socially constructed (Lawton 2000). Good (1994) makes a distinction between conditions that are easily rendered by the objectivist approach of medical science and other conditions such as pregnancy or chronic illness that are distorted by the rationalising medical gaze. Drawing on studies of chronic pain he argues that serious illness and pain provoke a transformation in the embodied experience of the life world. This perspective, however, has been challenged by writers who suggest it is based on simplistic assumptions about the status of the self prior to suffering an illness (Fox 2002). Bodily experiences and individual expressions of those experiences need to be placed in context. Sennett (1994) for example has argued that there is a strong link between the denial of bodily pain, the acknowledgement of pain and the material conditions of urban life.

While illness changes our bodies and personal biographies, New Medical Technologies (NMTs) and Enhancement Technologies (ETs) are changing our notions of the self, identity and bodily boundaries (Brown and Webster 2004; Hogle 2005). These new technologies are colonising and creating an increasing number of fields from telemedicine, electronic patient records, bio-informatics to pharmacogenomics. However, it would be wrong to see these developments in simplistic terms as just enabling new forms of power and surveillance to operate. If we consider technologies aimed at substituting the body, for example, there is a long history of people with disabilities interacting with technology. Current concerns with cyborgs may reflect a privileging of the exotic over the mundane. There are therefore patterns of continuity and discontinuity in NMT. Continuities are found in systems of classification and measurement, in the deepening of the medicalisation of the lifecourse and in the extension of individual choice. Discontinuities can equally be found in the increase in the diversity of existing socio-biological boundaries. For example, Brown and Webster (2004) suggest that images used in telemedicine become hyper-real leaving the patient in a disembodied limbo.

Anthropologists have shown that humans have always modified their bodies using various invasive techniques but Hogle (2005) suggests that the applications of new technologies to body enhancement are closely related to a shift in the nature of modernity. Whereas modernity had previously focused on improving social conditions through political and social institutions; new technologies offer opportunities for improvement at the level of individual bodies and personal taste. NMTs and ETs develop within a complex dynamic of social, legal, political, economic, medical and cultural responses to health and illness. The field is changing at a breathtaking rate as new technologies are continually being revised and developed to address new and existing needs and desires in what is an inter-related and dynamic process. One immediate consequence of this flux is that the boundary between what is agreed to be a therapeutic process and what constitutes an enhancement or cosmetic intervention becomes increasingly difficult to define and regulate. Anti-ageing medicine as we shall see in Chapter 6 is an area of particular controversy in this respect (Post and Binstock 2004). There are also strong commercial and demographic drivers to the pursuit of technologies addressing life extension, age specific illnesses and the appearance of ageing (Juengst *et al.* 2003). The capacity to alter one's appearance and delay the onset of ageing may however have only temporary effects, leading to a continual process of managing and monitoring the appearance of ageing.

The availability of new technologies offering bodily enhancement has repercussions across the lifecycle as they open up new ways of constructing social relations and social inequalities. Marshall (2002), for example, argues that successful ageing has incorporated notions of sexual functionality across the lifecourse so that erectile dysfunction has been promoted as a health problem with clear medical solutions. She suggests that this is leading to a new bodily configuration founded on the medicalisation of male sexuality and a social and political rejection of the late-life ageism of the past in favour of what she refers to as 'mid-life ageism' in the present. Indeed, there is some evidence to suggest that increasing emphasis on bodily appearance is shifting ageist attitudes down the age structure towards younger age groups (Sennett 2006).

Within second modernity previous institutional means of addressing individual well-being and welfare are increasing challenged by individualised medical responses offering the means of self-mastery and self-enhancement (Martin 2000). This also challenges existing understandings of citizenship as these are increasingly centred on the body as a means of maintaining and constructing identity (Hogle 2005). Shilling (1993) refers to this as a 'crisis of meaning' and draws on Haraway's (1991) work on the cyborg to highlight the opportunities and risks of new technologies and the way they force us to question continually what it now means to be human. Haraway herself has referred to a 'new world order' to describe the ways in which embodiment is becoming 'post-human' within the imperatives of global capitalism (Haraway 1997). Haraway is not the only one to view new technologies as offering opportunities and threats. Virtual reality as a technology now allows for a separation of body and experience so that the body becomes invisible and has thus been seen as a means of providing new ways of living and gaining autonomy for people with disabilities, older people and people with chronic illness. 'Disembodied encounters' in virtual worlds can conceal disability, reduce stigma and allow people experiences outside bodily limits. Featherstone (1991) discusses these possibilities with respect to ageing bodies and sees utopian and dystopian possibilities. Cyberspace may allow us to be free of bodily limits but is what it offers shallow and superficial? In particular, with respect to older people, instead of engaging in a society marked out by propinquity will it not be more tempting for individuals to occupy private spaces of virtual reality – to relive memories and to reconstruct dead friends and partners? It is also important to consider possible inequalities in access to these technologies (Brook 1998). Technologies may eventually address individual memories, regenerative medicine and even, according to the transhumanist movement, immortality through interfacing and downloading the brain to conscious-computers (see: www.terasemfoundation.org/) but the danger is that we are witnessing an expansion in the commodification of bodily forms and human relations being couched increasingly in terms of legalised property relations.

From the above discussion it should be clear that understandings of the body are historically and socially contingent (Shilling 1997, 2005). Indeed, the body as a single entity may be an illusion that is reconstructed and de-constructed across time and the existing dominant medical paradigm takes a key role in that process (Forth and Crozier 2005). For example, metaphors for the body reflect the dominant scientific and technical concerns of the day, from the mechanical metaphors that accompanied Descartes' mind–body split and the impact of Newtonian science through to the imagery of networks that has been a strong theme in modern bio-medical writing (Sontag 1989). Time and temporality are important here, as Newton (2003) suggests, because biologically based bodily processes may be subject to a slower pace of change thus putting bodies beyond social construction while simultaneously the cultural interpretation of the body is subject to a very rapid change. The notion of genetic causality and the capacity of MRI scans of the brain to account for personality differences are just two examples. This leads Newton to argue that the intertwining of biological and social aspects of the body presents difficulties for realist approaches that emphasise the enduring nature of structures. At the same time however, Newton has little sympathy for postmodern approaches to the body which appear to have a growing influence within the field of social gerontology.

Postmodern critiques and realist responses to the loss of meaning

Recent work addressing the body in gerontology has adopted post-modern perspectives to criticise the 'modernist' bio-medical dominance within gerontology and its emphasis on universal notions of the ageing body (Powell and Longino 2001). This critique is given a Foucauldian twist whereby the practices of bio-medicine and gerontology with respect to older bodies are constructed as part of a disciplinary and normalising gaze that reinforces existing power relations (Powell and Biggs 2000). Fox (2002) expresses dissatisfaction with a perceived tendency in the literature on the body to create a polarisation between on one side the privileging of subjective experience over social structure and on the other side rationalist bio-medical accounts of corporeality. In part this may reflect a division between medical sociology and social gerontology. The emphasis on subjective experience is common in studies of chronic illness and disability while the emphasis on a biological basis for ageing exists much more strongly within gerontology. While there have been moves within medical sociology away from subjectivist accounts towards a greater engagement with biology, equally social gerontology has witnessed movements to emphasise social construction in ageing. In response to these polarised accounts, Fox suggests a pragmatic approach combining essentialist lived experience with an accommodation of social context (Fox 1999). He draws extensively on Deleuze and Guattari's (1988) notion of embodiment where a 'self' is impossible without 'a body'. But here embodiment is always an unfinished project so that subjectivity is understood as a continual reworking of embodiment within socio-cultural structures. There are three strands to this approach to embodiment. First, the *Body without Organs (BwO)*, although a contested and ill-defined term, refers to the 'virtual' state of being apart from the organism and facing the fluidity and multiplicity of endless becoming. Second, *Territorialisation* refers to a process of dynamic interaction between psychic and social physical forces. For example, physicians de-territorialise patients through their bio-medical gaze and re-territorialise them with their bio-medical codes. Finally, *the nomadic subject* refers to absolute de-territorialisation of the *BwO* and *nomadology* refers to a multiplicity of narratives enabling a 'line of flight' away from traditional orthodox grand narratives allowing the postmodern self the potential freedom to roam and escape the limits of illness, disability and old age. Fox (2002) uses this framework to ask is it possible to nomadically refuse/resist the territory of health? Replacing the usual theoretical question of what constitutes a body with 'what can a body do?' he posits an active, engaged, open and experimenting body:

> For patients, people with disabilities, older adults and for anyone, the social may impinge to territorialize the BwO, to establish limits from which it is hard to fly. But these limits can be redrawn, especially if one has a little help.
>
> (Fox 2002: 359–60)

Unfortunately, while Fox's critique is interesting it does not escape a caricature of bio-medical thought with respect to the body and falls victim to a confusion of essentialism and determinism in rejecting an underlying biological reality. As Sayer (2000) argues, much anti-essentialist and postmodern thinking is based on two claims about modernist thought; its epistemological dogmatism leading to assertions of absolute truth and its ontological determinism leading to the view that people's lives, actions and relationships are determined by nature. A way out of this as Sayer goes on to argue, is to adopt a realist perspective, which bases knowledge claims on fallibilism; that is the view that all knowledge is contingent and fallible. When postmodernists question a claim to truth, such as a bio-medical view of the body, they are in fact inferring that something exists independently of this claim. To suggest that there are multiple and equally valid claims about human bodies is therefore contradictory. With respect to ontological determinism, we can argue that the essence of a thing is not the sum of its properties. While its essence constrains its activity it does not determine it and likewise to talk of human nature is not to imply determinism (Lawson 2003). Indeed, reference to the importance of the biological body does not imply a commitment to uniformity and static notions of embodiment. Burkitt (1999), for example, rejects the view of bodies as texts that do not exist extra linguistically but attempts to theorise a material body without losing the insights of the constructivist view. A realist approach to the body rejects fixed, norm-based and pathologised accounts of human bodies. As Soper (1995) has argued, claims of the oppression of female bodies, aged bodies, racialised bodies and the bodies of working class people become meaningless if they are based on a view of human bodies as cultural constructs or the free-floating products of textual play. Furthermore, the variety of bodily forms that human cultures are capable of can be legitimately postulated as being a consequence of a universal human nature giving a foundation to the critiques of the oppressive exercise of power and its impact on the bodies of particular groups or classes in society (Collier 2003). It is from this position that we suggest one should address the ageing body in the context of rapid social change. Is the biological body the essence of ageing or does society interact with these processes to create not only different ways of experiencing the ageing but maybe what constitutes the ageing body itself?

The reflexive self, the lived experience of disability and the vicissitudes of ageing bodies

As we have noted, several authors (Giddens 1991; Bauman 2000; Beck, Giddens and Lash 1994; Beck 2006) have argued that we are experiencing a period in history that has witnessed a decline in religious, political and social certainties. Traditional and modernist frameworks that once gave us a clear world-view have become subject to uncertainty and flux. Consequently, people are forced to seek individualised solutions to the problems of identity and this 'self-reflexivity' has become a social norm. Furthermore, such self-reflexivity is occurring at a time when not only are people living longer but developments in genetic engineering, biological reproduction and cosmetic surgery are promising individuals an increasing degree of control over their bodies. If we relate these developments to the criteria for understanding later life in the context of second modernity as described in Chapter 1 (Table 1) it may be possible to think about the body in later life in ways that bring fresh light to bear on the increasingly heterogeneous experience of ageing. For example, a study of older people in Sweden (Bullington 2006) examined responses to ageing and ageing bodies and identified three ideal types. The first, *'existential awakening'* was related to responses of shock, loss and awareness of death. Here the physical was less important than existential aspects of ageing. Respondents did not like their bodies, found them unattractive and tended to direct activity away from the self towards others. In the second type, *'making it good enough'*, respondents tended to focus on a changing body (good and bad), gave accounts of a battle between the self and body and rationalised ageing in terms of making best of the situation. The third type described as *'new possibilities'* were largely male, appeared 'at home' with their bodies, referred to the freedoms brought on by retirement and focused on future activities. Bullington concluded that the diverse experiences of the ageing body are related to changes in society that enable such choices to be made.

Where second modernity gives rise to a multiplying of social boundaries and institutional turbulence it seems likely that individual bodies and bodily surveillance will become sites for conflicts over categories of ageing. The emphasis within second modernity on different claims to knowledge becomes acute in relation to the growth of identity issues that are very much centred on bodily appearance, behaviour, and sexuality (Elliot and Lemert 2006). A crucial question for the study of later life therefore is the extent to which aged bodies lose or gain status within a 'social market' of identities. If, as some suggest, we are witnessing the birth of the 'quasi-subject' where reflexive individuals are expected to choose quickly from uncertain outcomes, as researchers, we need to ask what choices are available to older groups in society and whether and how do ageing bodies place limits on such choices? Equally, if ageing is occurring in the context of increasing individualisation, uncertain careers and unstable lifecourses, does this present the possibility of new inequalities arising based around the bodily appearance and bodily practices? Are the surface qualities of youthful appearance being privileged at the expense of age, memory and experience? Finally, in an increasingly insecure social order, do the vicissitudes of ageing bodies provide further disadvantage to older groups or are there new ways and opportunities for individuals to construct their own biographies and, as Fox (2002) argues, escape the 'limits' of their bodies?

How do these questions and insights aid and further our understanding of the lived experience of later life? One of the reasons the
body is central to the study of ageing is the increased likelihood of
experiencing chronic illness and disability as we enter later life (Hockey
and James 1993). A useful parallel may be the social model of disability which has dominated the field of disability studies for some
time and has had a profound influence over approaches to disability
and chronic illness (Barnes, Mercer and Shakespeare 1999; Zarb and
Oliver 1993). The parallel arises because of concerns about the role,
or lack of role, of the biological body in constructing the reality of
disability and the extent to which this could be applied to ageing.

The social model of disability makes a point of challenging what
are seen as individual models of disability where the disability is seen
in terms of a 'personal tragedy'. In contradistinction, advocates of the
social model see disability resulting from society rather than any
putative impairment. Indeed some influential disability theorists see no
link between impairment and disability at all (Oliver 1996). However,
it can be argued that while the body is at the heart of contemporary
political and theoretical debate, the social model of disability succeeds
only in removing the body from discussion (Hughes and Paterson 1997).
In the context of community care and social policy, for example, Twigg
(2002) has argued that the social gaze of the social worker renders the
body invisible despite community care being saturated by body-work.
In the process of building the case against the *social* oppression of
disabled people the body is generally ignored by advocates of the
social model of disability leaving the body invisible and at the mercy
of medicine. Artificial distinctions between medicine's reductive gaze
and nursing's holistic approach to bodies (Lawler 1997) do little to
address this problem. Best (2007) for example, asks whether a socially
constructed conception of pain is possible or desirable. Contrary to a
number of postmodern-inspired conceptions that pain exists exclu-
sively at the level of discourse and linguistic construction (Fox 2002),
pain needs to be viewed as a material barrier that exists beyond the
politico-aesthetic level. In a similar fashion for ageing the body is
much more than a canvas upon which we can create appropriate dis-
cursive formations to incorporate preferred identities. To recognise
the existence of biologically based realities is not to accept biological
dysfunction or decline as the sole cause of disability or indeed ageing.

In rejecting simplistic social constructionist accounts of the body
for ageing we also need to be aware of some of the insights that

disability theorists are able to bear on the issue of embodiment. Carol Thomas (2007), in her work on reconciling the different discourses brought into play by both disability studies and medical sociology, acknowledges that the social model of disability needs to situate the processes of disability within a sociology of the lived experience of people with disability and that this must include some discussion of the biological context of the various conditions. Instead of simply accepting the conflation of impairment with dysfunction and therefore disability, she instead offers the idea of 'impairment effects' which intermesh impairment with the social conditions that bring them into being and give them meaning. In this way bio-social relationships are embedded in impairment effects but are not reducible to them. In seeing opportunities for the development of a critical realist approach to disability studies Thomas is also providing inspiration for a similar approach to take root within studies of the ageing body. The too simple equation between age and impairment has not only been challenged by many of the demographic and epidemiological characteristics of contemporary ageing but also by the lived experiences of many of those entering later life. These cohorts have experienced the relationship between health, ageing and the body in different ways to preceding cohorts and it could be argued that they have created a bodily 'generational habitus' that reconfigures our understanding of what ageing and its vicissitudes may mean.

Conclusion

In this chapter we have reviewed some of the key theoretical approaches to the sociology of the body and their relevance to later life. As Twigg (2004) points out, the body is central to the understanding of ageing. Its significance can be found in the body's role in subjective experiences of ageing, in the experience of deep old age, in cultural representations of later life and in the ways in which care work is a form of body-work that is strongly gendered. However, beyond generalised statements about issues of decline and the inevitability of death (Elias 1985; Shilling 2005) there have been few serious engagements from those working within the sociology of the body on the topic of the ageing body. Even Wainwright and Turner's (2006) discussion of ageing ballet dancers would seem to be more about the peculiarities of professional dance than it is about ageing per se. A notable exception is the work of Simon Williams (2003) who in his

Medicine and the Body attempts to bring an understanding of the importance of ageing into a well rounded appreciation of corporeality. The work, however, of addressing some of the novel features of ageing has been left to a small number of what could be termed cultural gerontologists. Some writers have made inroads into creating a viable sociological basis for a cultural sociology of later life (Gilleard and Higgs 2000; Fairclough 2003) and the work of Gullette (2004) has highlighted the importance of culture in defining and regulating the aged body. Twigg, however, suggests that this is an area where research is in its infancy and bemoans the extent to which much of the existing literature is overly based on personal accounts of engagements with ageing bodies particularly in middle age. The body is key to understanding the boundaries between third and fourth ages and body failure. Lawton (1998) argues that western society is 'intolerant' of bodily failures many of which are equated with ageing and it is this fact that makes it a crucial topic in any sociology of the body. It is also one of the key areas of distinction for understanding the relationship between the biological nature of ageing and its social context. We can take this point further by suggesting that, in the context of second modernity, there is a heightened emphasis on individualised active ageing, the will to health, choice and the quasi-subject all of which have a direct relationship with the realities of the ageing body. Only where resources, both financial and cultural, are available, will there be opportunities for the perceived limits to the body to be challenged, questioned and transcended. As with many opportunities offered by changing circumstances, there is always the danger that these same circumstances may also expose bodily decay and decline and therefore risk being taken as signs of personal failure and lack as much as of success. It is in these changed circumstances that the somatic society becomes an important feature of later life.

4 New developments in social gerontology

Introduction

This chapter examines recent developments in social gerontology and considers the extent to which social transformations in the late twentieth century and early twenty-first century require a re-thinking of a sociology of old age (Phillipson 1998; Vincent 1999). The impact of a globalised society has different impacts on older people depending on their social and geographical location. The decline of traditional welfare support mechanisms may mean that the less affluent will experience inequalities in material and cultural terms, while the affluent face a future of multiple identities of choice based on their capacity to participate in global consumption networks (Gilleard and Higgs 2000). These networks draw strength from the exploitative relations of untrammelled global capitalism (Beck 2005). While cohorts of older people face uncertainty in retirement as winners or losers in the pensions lottery, the pension funds they have little or no control over have become the big players in determining future global flows of capital (Blackburn 2002). Discussing advances in critical gerontology, feminist gerontology and postmodern gerontology in turn, the chapter will look at how these different theoretical positions provide insights into the ways in which radical transformations in social life are giving rise to profoundly different experiences of later life.

Globalised society and old age

As the experience of old age becomes a norm for people in the developed and developing world (HelpAge International 2002) so the ageing of populations becomes a contemporary social and political challenge at the global level (Palacios 2002). However, processes of demographic ageing are uneven. Older, mostly richer, countries face threats from an increase in the ratio of older to working age people. As Palacios points out this manifests itself financially in two ways, first directly through impacts on pension and health programmes and second indirectly through impacts on productivity levels. Poorer countries on the other hand face the prospect of becoming old before becoming rich. Around two-thirds of the world's older people live in developing countries and while the number of older people tripled in the last half of the twentieth century this number is expected to triple again, reaching 2 billion by 2050 (United Nations 2002).

As Harper (2006) argues, forecasting population growth, levels of fertility and dependency is an uncertain business and scenarios for developed and developing countries cover a range of possible trends. Nevertheless, as rates of child mortality decline and mortality in young adults falls, it is likely that the general pattern will be one of a convergence in fertility and mortality rates between the developed and less developed countries by the middle of this century (United Nations 2002). Ageing in less developed countries will have uncertain effects and is related to levels of poverty in these countries (Gutierrez-Robledo 2002). There are potential benefits from having more stable population profiles and a larger population of older people. However, the speed of demographic ageing in developing countries in the context of high levels of lifetime absolute poverty means that many countries are poorly prepared for the impact of future ageing (HAI 1999). In terms of the health of older people in developing countries there are three clear areas concern; (i) the rising burden of caring as a result of high rates of HIV related deaths, (ii) traditional extended family safety nets have been weakened, (iii) older people are becoming the principal breadwinners and care givers for young children orphaned through HIV related mortality.

Globalisation is a highly contested term but most would agree that the concept refers to expansions in the magnitude, scale, speed and impact of transborder activities across the world (Held *et al.* 1999; Held 2004). Shifts from organised to disorganised forms of capitalism (Lash and Urry 1987) and in forms of Welfare (Offe 1985; Esping-Andersen 2000) are key areas where transformation has occurred. These changes have been accompanied by new forms of risk and work (Beck 2005) and social relations (Giddens 1991), and such changes have transformed the lifecourse (Warnes 2006). In response

Estes and Phillipson (2002) argue that global transformations have given rise to a new political economy that is shaping the lives of older people. They characterise this in terms of shifts from the definition and regulation of old age through mass institutions in the post-Second-World-War period up to the 1970s to the more individualised and privatised structures of the present. These arguments tend to frame the postwar welfare consensus as an intergenerational contract based on solidarity (Walker 1981) that broke down following the crisis of the 1970s and subsequent rise of the New Right. The contradictions of the welfare state (Gough 1979) were picked up by gerontologists who argued that the welfare state constructed dependency in old age. However in the late twentieth century the institutions of welfare have changed and in changing have led to further problematisation of old age. A key component of Estes and Phillipson's (2002) critique is what they describe as the neo-liberal ideology at the heart of globalisation. While this is by no means an original statement (Harvey 2005), it represents a general redirection within critical gerontology away from previous statist accounts of political economy towards giving more attention to the impact of globalisation on later life (Baars *et al.* 2006). As the fluidity and speed of global capital flows places greater strains on the capacity of individual states to respond to global economic forces, they suggest neo-liberal ideology reinforces these trends by denigrating the role of states in regulating and managing global markets. As Bass (2006) points out however, there is an absence of adequate theorising in the gerontological literature about these developments, an absence which he thinks is exacerbated by gerontologists having a tendency to flag up key theorists without developing their relevance to the understanding of transformations in later life and relations between the welfare state and older members of society.

In examining the impact of globalisation it is important to distinguish between 'race to the bottom' or 'pessimist' theorists and those who see global processes as being more benign (Giddens 2000). We need empirical evidence of the effects of these global transformations on healthcare spending on older people, on pensions and incomes in old age and consumption patterns in later life (Mishra 1999; Blackburn 2002). The drive towards commodification and privatisation of later life, over the last decade in particular, is most clearly seen in the World Bank's emphasis on promoting private pension arrangements wherever possible (World Bank 1994). The World Bank's approach to social protection and pensions in developing countries is based on a multi-pillar framework composed of: (i) a non-contributory 'zero' pillar providing minimal protection, (ii) a first pillar linked to earnings, (iii) a mandatory second pillar based on individual savings, (iv) a voluntary third pillar and (v) informal intergenerational and intra-family resource transfers thought to reflect traditional forms of aged care in developing countries (World Bank 2005). The policies they advocate reflect a modification of previously more aggressive proposals leaving pension and elderly care low on the list of investment priorities and are in stark contrast to International Labour Organisation arguments for more universalist tax-based approaches to social protection in developing countries (Cichon 2004).

In the provision of health and social care it is also important to note that services for older people may be particularly vulnerable to marketisation; witness the dramatic increase in private homes for the elderly in the UK over the last 20 years where the blurred boundaries between nursing care and social care have been particularly open to exploitation and discrimination (Scourfield 2007). The promotion of a 'choice' agenda within UK health services may also have sharper consequences for the provision of healthcare for the elderly in two key respects. First, critics of the emphasis on choice point out that there are real dangers for some services where the outcome may not necessarily be the anticipated one of competition on the basis of quality of services but rather competition on the basis of price and cost with unintended consequences in terms of reductions in the quality of publicly funded services (Phillips 2007). Second, where resources are scarce and rationing occurs the 'choice' may be framed as one that is made between the interests of competing generations. Such distinctions could provide legitimacy to rationing by age or proxies for age (Fitzpatrick 2001). The increasing emphasis on the individualised subject, personal responsibility for health and well-being, as well as the transformation of welfare states from those based around universal provision into those based around governmentality may have particularly negative effects on those generations who contributed to the construction of traditional welfare state forms (Clarke, Smith and Vidler 2005).

Jane Lewis (2007) argues that European welfare systems have shifted away from a male breadwinner family model to an 'adult worker family model' where the emphasis is on productivism and labour market participation for both men and women. This move potentially exacerbates gender inequality in later life (Ginn 2003) and contributes to problems of inter-generational transfers of wealth (Kotlikoff 2003). The last forty years have witnessed significant changes in family forms, in labour market participation and in welfare policies. More women are in work (albeit a large proportion of them in part-time jobs and still on relatively lower pay than men). There has been a decline in male participation through redundancy and early retirement. Women's financial contribution to household incomes has gone up but this has not been accompanied by a change in the balance of unpaid work in the household (Gershuny 2000). At the same time family forms have become more fluid and there has been a rise in the divorce rate, family separation, cohabitation and single person households. Life-courses have become de-institutionalised, messy and complex. While patterns of work and household formation have changed, the Welfare state has experienced considerable restructuring around the welfare to work model. At the European level the emphasis in the twenty-first century is on work and productivism as a means of supporting welfare needs (European Commission 2000). This assumes that all adults, both male and female, participate in the labour market. Lewis (2007) refers to this as a 'new social settlement' and warns that it may have disastrous consequences for women in old age because of the burden of informal and formal care. Her argument is based on the view that the old male breadwinner model was based on two separate but related settlements, the first being between labour and capital where the glue was the guarantee of social insurance, the second being between the genders where female economic dependency was linked to care of the young and old. While the move towards the adult worker family model has accelerated, the unequal division of unpaid care work remains and acts as a barrier to women fully participating as citizen workers. Furthermore, the pressure from welfare state policies is for care to become defamilialised and commodified. But this creates problems in the private sphere of caring. The shift in welfare policies is based on an assumption of an increasingly individualised subject and the emphasis on rights and responsibilities, with a move away from welfare forms that emphasise social support, de-commodification and universal benefits to forms that focus on social inclusion, commodification and conditional often punitive benefit systems (Gilbert 2002). With respect to caring these trends ignore care that is based on reciprocity and emotional ties and the intrinsic, difficult to measure, aspects of caring are further devalued through processes of marketisation.

The crisis of welfare projected to arise from the demographic 'time bomb' may be overstated (Gee 2000). John Hills (2004) for example, maintains that predicting the impact of ageing populations is complex and increasing costs in one area of public spending may be offset by decreasing costs and increasing revenues in other areas. He concludes that although the pressures from an ageing population are upwards, 'they are taking place over a long period, and could be accommodated if we chose to do so' (Hills 2004: 246). It may be therefore that accounts of the decline of welfare provision are exaggerated. As a consequence more dangerous threats are ignored, including the impact of labour market instability, global recession, mass migration and political conflict. Moreover adaptation rather than downsizing of regimes of welfare may be the necessary response to such threats (Castles 2002). In these circumstances financial globalisation may ultimately lead to an expansion in modes of corporate governance driven by the power of large financial trusts including pensions funds (O'Sullivan 2000). In developed western countries the welfare state reform is linked to population ageing, family instability and changing labour market dynamics. As we have seen, attempts to adapt welfare systems have focused on privatisation, decentralisation and familialisation but welfare systems still face uncertainty and financial difficulty. For some, the generational inequality that accompanied the shift from a golden age to a silver age of welfare (Taylor-Gooby 2002) requires a re-orientating of policy priorities toward investment in constructing opportunities for younger generations (Esping-Andersen 2000). Many of today's pensioners enjoy a financial security unheard of for the generation that preceded them. This suggests, according to Myles (2002), the need for a new generational contract. These arguments are reflected in proposals from influential social democrat policy analysts at the heart of the EU which have generated considerable controversy (Esping-Andersen 2002). These involve the explicit introduction of 'intergenerational risk taking' into the financing of pensions and accept the need to control the costs of today's older population to make it acceptable for those retiring in the future. This is to be done by setting net benefits at a constant ratio to per capita earnings and thus ensuring that both worker and retired have an interest in the economic success of their nations. The welfare state which initially set itself the task of protecting the retiree from the vagaries of the market is now moving to fully integrate the market into the lives of pensioners (Esping-Andersen 2002).

Critical gerontology

The circumstances experienced by older people have often been seen as prompting the need for radical solutions. In response to the idea of old age being simply a category of social administration, researchers such as Peter Townsend (1981) introduced the idea of 'structured dependency' with its attendant ideas of regaining full citizenship rights. Critical gerontology emerged from these radical impulses. Phillipson (2003) concurs with this view of critical gerontology by seeing it as connected to earlier materialist if not neo-Marxist antecedents in the field of social policy. Drawing on materialist accounts where class, gender and race or ethnicity were seen as primary points of conflict and division in society, critical gerontology starts with an awareness of structural constraints. This forms the first pillar of critical gerontology. The second pillar is based on humanistic approaches that focus on the meanings associated with old age and underpinned by biographical approaches to later life. Finally, the third pillar is its aspirational aspect that focuses on the empowerment of older people. These three pillars come together to create a paradigm where ageing is socially constructed in and through the structures of the state and capital and in and through individual and group social relations.

The term critical gerontology therefore encompasses a range of theoretical interests often brought together with little concern for potential contradictions provided there is an overarching commitment to the social construction of ageing and opposition to positivist, naturalist and biologically driven notions of ageing (Baars 1991). Perhaps the strongest stream within critical gerontology has been that of the political economy approach (Estes 1979, 1986; Walker 1981) but there are differences between those working within a neo-Marxist paradigm, who emphasise the constraints exercised on human agency in old age and across the lifecourse by the structures and power relations of the capitalist economy (Estes 1986), and those working within a Weberian framework who balance the economic imperative with a recognition of the influence of state activities on the conditions of later life (Myles 1989). Others have been influenced by the German philosopher Jurgen Habermas' work and take a more nuanced approach to criticisms of the objectification of age and the lifecourse within mainstream gerontology (Moody 1993). Critics of the political economy of ageing approach have argued that it (i) potentially over-states structural constraints on individual agency and is economically deterministic and (ii) is unable to address evidence of high levels of affluence and well-being among large segments of the older popula-tion (Gilleard and Higgs 2000). In addition, the political economy approach has not kept up to date with developments in the welfare state or within theoretical accounts of these changes. This is ironic given that within mainstream social policy there are clear attempts to address changes in welfare state forms and theories of welfare at global levels (Gough 2004). But the relationship of class, welfare state and later life has not received the attention that it should have. Many of the changes to the funding of people in retirement, particularly in the Anglo-Saxon world, have moved retirees out of their 'de-commodified' status and have in effect 're-commodified' by making them more dependent upon the state of global financial markets[1]. All of this suggests that there needs to be a re-analysis of older people's rela-tionship to class rather than just treating them as determined by their previous positions in the class system (Higgs and Gilleard 2006).

Moving away from structured dependency theory and the political economy approach and taking on board some of the points made by Gilleard and Higgs (2000), Phillipson (2003) now recognises that later life has become a phase in the lifecycle open to individual negotiation rather than one controlled and defined by institutions of the state. The problem for a significant number of older people is that they lack the resources both in economic and social capital that allow them to negotiate this increasingly privatised sphere. The threats to vulnerable groups from individualisation are considerable. The shifting of bur-dens of care from society to individuals (particularly older women), as Hagestad and Dannefer (2001) point out, reflects an increasingly individualised gaze within gerontology itself that privileges a problem-oriented, bio-medical and personality-based response to the problems of later life. These changes have stimulated calls for an international approach to the political economy of ageing to address the challenges of neo-liberal global economic forms (Walker 2005). Again, however, the conceptual tools do not seem to be up to the task given that most critical gerontologists are still wedded to the idea that later life is still determined by the policies of individual welfare states and assumes that globalisation can only be problematic for older people (Polivka 2001). As mentioned previously, Zygmunt Bauman (1998) in his book on globalisation describes a world increasingly made up of 'tourists' who can experience the world without restrictions and 'vagabonds' who are bound to stay where they live for fear that they may become economic migrants. This division between the globals and the locals reflects the differential impact of globalisation and has much to say about the circumstances of older people throughout the modern world. At the most prosaic level this can be seen in terms of just who makes up those tourists and where they come from. Research examining the spend on tourism and flying indicates that in countries like Canada it is those over 50 who are increasing their spending on these activities and, surprisingly this is likely to be reflected in countries such as China who are entering the tourism market in a big way (Tretheway and Mak 2005).

In the USA and Canada there is already an established seasonal migration of older North Americans to warmer climates. This adds an extra dimension to the planning of services for older people in states such as Florida and Arizona where many of them go (Longino 1988), as well as Canadian nationals who are circumscribed regarding the amount of time that they can spend in another country without losing entitlements (Katz 2005). While this may seem to be a particularly North American problem, it is now something that affects Europe with large numbers of older EU citizens choosing to spend parts of the year in countries other than their own (King, Warnes and Williams 1998). This also brings new confusions to ideas of citizenship and national rootedness as was revealed in 2007 when 48,000 UK pensioners were paid an additional cold weather payment even though they did not live in the UK. Such complications mean that many of the assumptions used by the various strands of critical gerontology are in need of reconceptualising their starting points if they are to be more than anachronistic models of a world that has changed dramatically. Phillipson (2006) is aware that globalisation needs to be addressed in many new ways:

> Globalisation – as one constituent of the 'risk society' – will generate new forms of insecurity, of which anxieties and fears about ageing may represent a significant dimension. But other dimensions are less easy to predict: will a new cohort of older people (e.g. the post-war baby boom generation) give a different voice and meaning to the nature of growing old? If they do, to what extent will this be determined by social networks that

embrace global as well as local contexts? To what extent will globalisation undermine the social, economic and cultural threads
(tenuous at best given the role of class, gender and ethnicity) linking
together people identified through biological age? Globalisation
has certainly transformed the world but it is changing growing
old as well – and in equally radical ways.

(Phillipson 2006: 207)

Feminist gerontology

For a long time feminism and old age seemed to occupy separate
worlds. When Simone de Beauvoir wrote 'long before the eventual
mutilation, woman is haunted by the horror of growing old' (de
Beauvoir 1993 [1949]: 605–6) she was referring to the expectations
that women in French bourgeois society remained young and beauti-
ful. This overarching patriarchal imperative defined their and others'
views of old age and particularly of older women. In today's consumerist and celebrity-focused environment her words may be more
prescient than ever but they also presage a long-term ambivalence
within feminist thought towards later life and a lack of engagement
with old age. In the early 1970s within feminisms there were attempts
to address this perceived lack of attention regarding the situation of
older women (Lewis and Butler 1972). But feminist writers and
researchers remained largely silent on the issue of ageing. This situation persisted, despite a general awareness of differences in the patterning of health and mortality between men and women. It has been
established for some time that, in western developed countries at
least, older women are more likely to live in poverty and to have
poorer pension provision because of discontinuities in employment
across their lifecourse (Garner 1999; Ginn 2003). Furthermore, women
are more likely to shoulder the burden of caring for older people,
either informally as part of responsibilities of family and kinship or
formally as paid carers within health and social care settings (Arber
and Ginn 1995). Extending the political economy approach, recent
work on levels of wealth and health suggest gender differences may
be due to a combination of both women having differential exposure
to material wealth over their lifecourse *and* being more vulnerable to
lower levels of material wealth across their lives (Arber 2006; Denton
2007). Feminist ideas seem particularly suited to exploring the social
construction of later life, particularly in the ways feminist writers (from
different strands of feminist thought) articulate women's oppression

through capitalist structures that sustain and promote differences in gender roles and responsibilities. Feminism can expose the links between privatisation and policy concerns with supporting traditional family structures as well as the low economic value placed on gender based care of older people. Despite these facts and theoretical insights it was not until the early 1990s that gerontology and feminism came together in an explicit academic sense with periodic calls among scholars for feminist approaches to research ageing. For example, Calasanti and Zajicek (1993) argued for ageing to be studied in the context of socio-historical constructions of class, gender and racial relations while Ray (1999) presented arguments for more critical feminist approaches to gerontology. Calasanti (1999) has suggested that part of the problem may lie in the way that feminist research on ageing tends to be marginalised and excluded from mainstream gerontology and that there is an underlying assumption within gerontology that feminist theory and feminist approaches to research only apply to women. More recently, Calasanti (2004) has argued that feminist gerontology requires a long-term, often career-damaging, investment in reconceptualising research around intersecting power relations. These calls have to some extent been answered from different perspectives. Feminist approaches to political economy have been applied to the study of welfare to show how, in the USA, privatisation policies and neo-conservative ideology reinforce traditional patriarchal family structures (Estes 2004). One of the key influences on mainstream feminist thought has been that of Carol Gilligan's work on an ethics of care (Gilligan 1982). Using these ideas to criticise mainstream gerontology Lloyd (2004) argues that a conceptual framework based on an ethics of care provides a powerful counterbalance to the emphasis on independence, autonomy and citizenship to be found in contemporary social policy and social gerontology. Other streams of feminist thought have influenced approaches to ageing that focus on ageism and resistance to ageism. Echoing earlier work on the concept of the 'crone' (Walker 1985), Germaine Greer (1991) argued in favour of embracing the ageing process and the 'natural' limits of the menopause as a means of opening up new avenues for resisting the dominance of sexuality. These ideas remain a strong feature of feminist gerontology which seeks to resist hegemonic masculinity but also the possibility of ageist tendencies within feminist thought (Ray 2004) while others have suggested that conditions within post-industrial society have led to a de-gendering of later life (Silver 2003).

It seems therefore that despite the earlier ambivalence towards old age, feminist thought has made substantial and growing contributions towards understandings of later life. However, there are areas where overlap with medical sociology and debates within mainstream sociology may add to this contribution. For example, sociologists in recent years have focused on changes in gender roles in the context of changes to labour market structures and class relations. Hakim (2000) has argued that the contraceptive revolution of the 1960s and the equal opportunities revolution of the 1970s transformed women's lives and expanded the choices available to them and goes so far as to argue that lifestyle preferences have become more important as determinants of social location than sex and gender (Hakim 2007). Others maintain that the structural constraints on women's lives still have a profound effect on their life chances (Crompton and Lyonette 2005). One thing however is clear. The social transformations that occurred from the early 1960s onwards were fought for and experienced by women who are now entering later life. In order to understand their experiences of ageing we need a research framework that takes account of the period and cohort effects that contextualise their lifecourses.

In the parallel field of medical sociology, feminism and feminist research has had a considerable influence on the choice of research fields, on approaches to research methodology and on participatory research (Bell 1992). As Macintyre and colleagues point out (Macintyre, Hunt and Sweeting 1996) gender differences in health, particularly within social epidemiology, tend to be presented in oversimplified ways leading to overgeneralisations of simple male/female differences across time, space and culture. This occurs despite the available evidence showing more complex and nuanced relationships between gender and health. Many have bemoaned the lack of historical context to much research addressing gender and health, arguing that there is a need to examine the mechanisms that connect changes in the gender order to changes in the experience of health and illness (Annandale and Hunt 2000). Where researchers have adopted more historic and contextualised approaches to the study of gender and health they have made considerable advances in our understanding of later life. For example, Hunt (2002) has demonstrated, using data from the West of Scotland twenty-07 study, that there are profound differences in the experiences, opportunities and attitudes of women born in the early 1930s compared to those born in the 1950s; she relates this to the substantial changes in gender relations that occurred in the second half of the twentieth century.

The significance of feminist gerontology for social gerontology as a whole has been summarised by Simon Biggs (2004) as allowing for a rapprochement between those who see age inequality in terms of structure and those who have examined the experiences of ageing in an ageist society. In particular, Biggs sees the value of examining issues of identity and performativity which have been underplayed in critical gerontological thinking but which have played an important role in much feminist theorising. Taking these insights further then leads to the possibility that studies of ageing can start to engage with the contested nature of the identities people adopt as they age as well as being aware of the temporal dimension of individual narratives of self.

Postmodern gerontology

Any movement towards the topic of identity inevitably moves into the intellectual terrain of postmodernism. As conventional distinctions of class, gender and race are challenged both in terms of their sociological categorisation and in terms of their salience for understanding contemporary social life, a whole host of new positions have emerged based on this relative indeterminacy. Many writers have seen postmodernism as offering new opportunities for freedom, choice and openness (Smart 1993). Following on from this, some postmodern gerontologists have identified that, under these new circumstances, age could be released from the negative status that currently blights it and ageing identities could be constructed and reconstructed in playful and self-conscious ways (Murphy and Longino 1997; Wilson 1997). Featherstone and Hepworth (1998) repeat this optimistic theme seeing the rise of new medical technologies as means of extending youthfulness and opening new doors of opportunity for older people to engage in lifestyles of choice (at least those old people with the resources to do so). Within this scenario agency becomes increasingly important as people are freed from the constraints of traditional institutional lifecourses as well as previous cultural expectations of ageing by new bio-technologies, information technologies and rising affluence. From this point of view postmodernity is not something to be feared, rather its combination of post-human technology and culture offers the means to free older people from 'naturalistic' notions of biological ageing. Ageing is thus conceived as multilayered and plastic with 'old age' becoming almost meaningless. Baudrillard (1993), the doyen of postmodern thought certainly believed that old age had increasingly become an identity of 'not age'. He also went on to point out that avoiding being identified with old age was just one of many identities that could be adopted. In these circumstances the fear of becoming old or of dying does not disappear but these fears take on different forms. They become the fears associated with the loss of identity, the loss of choice and a decline in creativity and self-expression. Such a position is a long way away from mainstream social gerontology. For Phillipson there is a fear that postmodern society lacks the core features that enable the maintenance of a viable identity for living in old age (Phillipson 1998); and Polivka (2000) views the hyper-individualism of the postmodern cyber-culture as precipitating a decline in spirituality, solidarity and support for welfare systems. It is very much the case that postmodernism thrives on the superabundance of signifiers within contemporary post-scarcity environments and in doing so raises culture and agency above the economic and structural. The question for the study of ageing is the degree to which postmodernism adequately describes the social changes experienced over the last half century and the extent to which the opportunities for free expression that Featherstone and Hepworth highlight may be restricted to those with the wealth to purchase them.

The cultural turn in gerontology

If postmodernism in social gerontology offers a too indeterminate reading of the status of later life in the modern world, it has none the less opened up social gerontology to a wealth of other strands that have been previously downplayed. This is not to say that the cultural dimension has been absent from research on ageing as the work by Gubrium and Holstein (2002) and Stephen Katz (2005) among a host of others demonstrates. However the recent interest in the issues of lifestyle (Cruikshank 2003), health (Lock 1993) and identity (Gullette 2004) has led to a resurgence of thinking about the relation between later life and the cultural forms in which it is lived out. A recurring issue for these writers is that of age identity and how it connects with an ageist culture. As we have noted this has been picked up by feminist writers who are concerned about the gendering of old age and its meanings. Simon Biggs (1999), from an explicitly psychodynamic perspective, adopts Katherine Woodward's (1991) use of the term 'masquerade' to describe the process where the older person may be acting out a 'masque' of youthfulness as a way of avoiding the consequences of ageing in an ageist society. The term masquerade is used because the older person, in adopting these practices, draws attention to the presence of the very ageing that is being concealed. Unlike Featherstone and Hepworth's (1991) concept of the 'Mask of Ageing' wherein older people saw their ageing bodies as different from their inner self, Biggs' *The Mature Imagination* (1999) does not see the masquerade as simply a process of deception but rather a coping measure where the older adult is able to create a degree of internal psychological stability by being able to control social expectations about appropriate behaviours as well as perform a particular identity which may differ from an internal identity. While it is not necessary to accept all of the psychological reasoning behind this position, what is useful is that it is drawing attention to the way that ageing has to be negotiated and is negotiated in the context of an ageist society.

While for many, identity seems the province of postmodern thinking its effects are important to how later life is experienced in a second modernity. Shifting away from the postmodern playfulness of identity construction or psychodynamic theorising we would argue that in engaging with the tasks of identity construction in later life, retired people are not just adopting another 'non age' identity, but that they are also resisting a move to a void status. In *Identity* (2004) Bauman makes this clear by pointing out that while most of the population exist in a situation defined by the instability of identity, there are those who are not allowed the right to claim an identity at all: in his words an underclass. While Bauman is thinking about the status of refugees and the '*sans papiers*', it is possible to see physically and mentally frail older people as also falling into this category. They exist on the other side of a cultural and policy divide. The oldest 'old' find that their identity is submerged into their health status and they have few resources (or capacities) to pursue their own identities. Moreover their needs are assessed and met by others deemed more competent. Not only do they lose the power of agency but they also become members of an ascribed community of fourth agers; the twenty-first century equivalents of the aged paupers of the workhouse. Even for those lucky enough to keep their distance from such identity hazards, the fear of falling into that category remains one of the key lines of fracture in later life (Gilleard and Higgs 1998).

In this way identity and agency in later life are bound together in ways that they were not in classical modernity where the ascribed identity of being old had purchase if not purchasing power. The lack of agency of the old was also matched by the relative lack of agency of other ascribed identities in the population such as worker, wife or unemployed. If identity construction in later life is now part of the process of growing older then it does matter whether the identity is chosen or ascribed. Later life and the identities within it need to be seen as constructed around agency and the validity of an agentic third age (Gilleard and Higgs 2005). The identity of simply being old no longer has force except in relation to the dependency of a 'fourth age' of decline and death.

This issue of identity also connects to another key concept in contemporary life, that of community. Again in the past the idea of community, fuzzy and ambiguous as it was, suggested a community of interest and interconnectedness of all age groups. Such communities were seen as natural and organic and their decline has been much discussed in the literature on social capital (Putnam 2000). Communities of identity are radically different, being marked out by their difference rather than their propinquity (Seidman 1997). In this world of difference and diversity the threat of being ascribed as old is one that is often resisted and in part accounts for the relative failure of age-based movements. The notion of older people as a community of identity is one that is hard to popularise because even for older people the ascribed status of old age is one without power with too many connections to frailty and dependency. Policies and services most obviously aimed at the old are those generally most resisted by the people for whom they are intended. In such ways are the body, ageing and identity now connected to social policy and politics.

Conclusion

This chapter has considered the consequences of recent social changes at a global level for later life. It has examined the transformation of traditional notions of welfare with respect to old age and shown how many of the conventional models used in social gerontology have needed to adapt to cope with the consequences of these changes. However these difficulties have also had the effect of allowing new paradigms such as feminism and postmodernism to provide fresh insights into the study of later life. A crucial concept that has emerged out of this engagement is that of identity which when related to ageing and old age has considerable purchase in describing many of the features of contemporary ageing often missing from mainstream accounts. We also drew attention to the significance of the cultural turn in social gerontology. This suggests a new agenda for research in social gerontology by focusing on the lived experience of ageing within contemporary societies. However, it also important to realise that we are in conditions of seeming rapid change and therefore we also need to constantly clarify our theoretical approaches to later life in a way that takes account of the period and cohort effects that contextualise old age.

5   The death of old age, critical approaches as undertakers

Introduction

It is possible to argue that sociology has avoided old age while old age is creeping up on sociology. Equally, the traditional subject matter of social gerontology may become less visible as ageing becomes more pervasive while at the same time its boundaries become less distinct. This chapter will address the changing features of old age and how it impacts on social gerontology. In particular it will examine the extent to which old age can be said to be dying out whether because of the impact of 'anti-ageing techniques', 'aspirational medicine' or the 'longevity revolution'. All of these topics appear to make later life as much a field for beauticians and plastic surgeons as it is for geriatric nurses and geriatricians.

The significance of bodily ageing is at the core of gerontology as well as of the challenges to it. What was taken as normative and unexceptional is now being re-articulated both in terms of culture and in terms of social relationships. Gilleard and Higgs (2000) break these changes into the following categories: *bodily appearance* which covers those cultural practices that shape and control age-associated changes in appearance; *bodily functioning* which examines changes in the 'machinery' of the body; and lastly *bodily control* where issues surrounding the individual's loss of the capacity for 'self care' are considered in the light of the civilised body.

Using these categories we can see how social gerontology has left relatively unchallenged many of the assumptions on which bio-ageing is based. This not only leads, as we have seen, to a lack of engagement with the burgeoning sociology of the body but also underplays the significance of agentic embodiment and its connection with consumer society. As Sulkunen (1997) points out:

The issue of the social constitution of the body is important in consumer society because everything we consume is taken in, enjoyed and processed by the body, whether through the tactile senses of touch taste and smell, or through the distant senses of the eye and the ear.

(Sulkunen 1997: 6)

The ageing of the body correspondingly plays a key role in connecting corporeality to consumption given that it is the fear of bodily ageing that permeates much of contemporary culture, boosting the sales of a wide variety of products ranging from anti-ageing cosmetics to vitamin supplements. The significance of ageing is not confined to the commodification of individual fears and desires. Concerns about the 'greying' of the population also permeate the mass media. At the level of public discourse, age-related bodily decline is not important because of its impact on how people look but because the desire to avoid or resist decline drives the growing lifestyle aspirations of young and old alike. In this way the two issues of avoiding the onset of ageing and the prevention of costly age-related morbidity have become important aspects of people's lives. To use Bauman's terminology – looking after your body as well as preventing or putting off a costly old age are important 'postmodern' virtues in the aestheticisation of everyday life (Bauman 1995).

In addition to these individual and social concerns about bodily ageing there is also a growing problematisation of what constitutes the normal body and what constitutes the ageing process. This uncertainty is expressed in various ways. Developments in medical technology have radically transformed what can be done to the body; skin grafts, organ transplants, bio-mechanical prostheses, etc. (Featherstone and Hepworth 1998). What can be expected and at what age expectations are appropriately addressed has been thrown into confusion. The body has taken on a more plastic quality as fashion plays an increasing role in determining bodily physique. In these new circumstances physical appearance is projected as seemingly a matter of individual consumer action rather than the incidental consequences arising from working life. Challenging 'wholesome tastes', the physical stereotypes of masculinity and femininity, and foundationalist ideas of beauty, a growing range of bodily types compete as aesthetic models for the human form (Pitts 2003; Shilling 2005).

For these reasons, the rise of consumerism, the growing cultural salience of age and the increased uncertainty surrounding the nature of bodies, the understanding of ageing has been rendered problematic. The ageing body continues to play a critical role in determining the subject matter of gerontology but that role has been transformed in the circumstances of the twenty-first century.

Bodily appearance

The connection between ageing and the signs of ageing seems clear cut with old age being the manifestation of the ageing process and bodily decline. Certainly within biological gerontology the ageing body has been a central reference point from which to study and understand 'the ageing process' which is best defined by an increasing risk of irremediable physical disability and death (Medina 1996). While the age and duration of this period may differ and be subject to social and environmental factors, what it does suggest is that in the end age itself is unfair and creates greater disadvantage than that created by social inequalities. In the end age may be the great leveller. As we have seen earlier such foundationalist assertions cause difficulties for 'social constructionist' social gerontologists whose accounts of old age as a product of social processes have to take account of this biological finitude. This view is accepted by Kathleen Woodward (1991) who writes 'As we approach the extremity of old age we approach in the West the limit of the pure cultural construction of aging' (Woodward 1991: 194). Others including Kontos (1999) and Twigg (2000, 2006) have also concluded that the verities of a fourth age have been ignored by social constructionist approaches to ageing.

While this may be true, such conclusions run the risk of refocusing the gerontological gaze back on to an ageing of decline and disability and thereby avoiding an engagement with many of the significant changes occurring in the cultural dynamics of ageing. A variety of surgical and non-surgical anti-ageing cosmetic practices have become mainstream aspects of contemporary life not only in Europe and North America but in Asia and Latin America. While the rationales and practices may be controversial and seen as embodying patriarchal attitudes (Jeffreys 2005), what cannot be challenged is that anti-ageing has become a significant element in the discourse of ageing in contemporary societies. Not funded within either taxation-based or insurance-based healthcare systems, anti-ageing medicine remains very much a private business. Nevertheless, the rising popularity of cosmetic surgery has more than merely iconic value in demonstrating the plasticity of the ageing body. That a significant minority of people – usually those with the necessary material resources – do choose to have aesthetic surgery to rejuvenate their appearance shows what the many without those resources might also do had they similar opportunities. Much of the work of cosmetic surgeons concentrates upon 'anti-ageing' (or youth-enhancing) procedures. These are becoming more various and more technically sophisticated year on year. Current practices such as chemical skin peels, facelifts and tummy tucks are being constantly added to as new techniques are developed to further advance aesthetic solutions to the imperfections of bodily ageing. These developments are driven by market forces particularly operating within the baby boomer generation. What is surprising is that 'anti-ageing' cosmetic surgery is sought not only by people in their forties, fifties and sixties – the long middle ages – but also by noticeable numbers of people in their twenties and thirties. It seems probable that these cohort effects will persist, and cosmetic surgery and related procedures will become part of everyday life, providing more people with the potential to mould their appearance as they would like it to be. While it might be objected that skin peels, tummy tucks, forehead lifts and botox injections are only concerned with the surface plane of 'signification' and do not affect the fundamentals of biological ageing, it is not sufficient to regard anti-ageing cosmetic surgery as merely a cultural epiphenomenon of consumer culture. Equally it is not possible to dismiss the culture that surrounds anti-ageing techniques as simply being one of 'false consciousness' or 'bad faith'. The processes go much deeper and relate to the aestheticisation of both lifestyle and the body and are constitutive of modern life itself (Ransome 2005; Sassatelli 2007). Consequently while anti-ageing techniques do not 'restore' a youthful appearance they do reduce some of the 'un-aesthetic' aspects of ageing and thus play a similar role in society to fashion, hairstyle and body shape. Downplaying such cultural dimensions not only ignores important facets of society but also commits the anti-naturalistic fallacy of assuming that the world is as theoretical accounts would have it.

However, while anti-ageing techniques seem to challenge the inevitability of ageing, they do so by producing a new set of dilemmas centred around the decision about when to 'get out of' the market. The growing individualisation of the ageing experience suggests that such decisions will create distinctions amongst third agers, between those who, according to Gilleard and Higgs (2000), adopt a 'managed ageing' strategy and those opting for strategies of 'lifelong prolongevity'. Other anti-ageing technologies offer a more direct route toward preventing or delaying bio-ageing. Continuing medical research into various steroids, steroid-like compounds, vitamins and related nutrients seeks to gain small but measurable benefits in later life disease prevention. While cosmetic surgery exploits the possibilities of surgical technology to re-aestheticise the ageing body through a defined set of procedures, it remains a private and risky enterprise. Consumption of over-the-counter medicines and all the various 'anti-ageing' cosmeceuticals and nutraceuticals offers a less risky strategy but requires sustained lifestyle changes with little obvious benefit to show for them. Both practices nevertheless represent the active choices of consumers.

To these approaches must be added the field of 'anti-ageing medicine' which seeks to represent itself as a continuing part of medicine's modernist 'triumph over nature'. The range and scope of prophylactic high technology surgery is a small but significant component of a largely private healthcare industry that actively promotes itself as 'anti-ageing medicine'. A flavour of the approach can be gleaned in the following quote from the first issue of the journal *Anti-Aging Medicine*:

> A minimum of 40,000 lifespans [will be] extended annually by eliminating heart failure by a combination of medical options: totally implantable artificial hearts, a modified heart assist device, xenograph transplant/repair or microtransplantation of fetal heart cells in devitalized heart tissue … A 30 year reversal in the aging process will be achieved by means of an implantable hormonal/pacemaker device to deliver a concentrated mixture of growth factors/hormones in cyclic rhythm to improve basic cellular function resulting in maintenance of bone density, muscle strength and overall cardiovascular fitness.
>
> (Klatz 1996: xiv)

As has been pointed out in the furious debate over the status of anti-ageing medicine that has gone on within biological gerontology, the evidence base for such practices is extremely limited and often rather tenuously linked to experimental gerontological research (see Olshansky, Hayflick and Carnes 2002). The claims of anti-ageing medicine can be seen as part of what Gilleard and Higgs have called 'aspirational science', a social construction which has flourished within postmodern scientific culture rather than a development of traditional 'modern medicine'. Indeed, the hostility to anti-ageing medicine by established figures such as James Fries and Leonard Hayflick has not just been seen as a form of boundary maintenance (Binstock 2004) but the hostility also emerges from writers who feel that anti-ageing medicine reinforces a particular form of 'ageism' that cannot accept the existence of an old age itself and therefore seeks to eliminate it (Vincent 2006a).

Bodily functioning

Physical ageing seems to occur autonomously, mainly outside the roles and resources that society does or does not provide for later life. As such, it imposes its own constraints on how later life can be lived and experienced. It implies a pattern that has to be adapted to, that cannot itself be fashioned. Yet evidence shows that access to the social and material resources of a society affects people's chances of survival and their likelihood of developing potentially disabling illnesses (McMunn *et al.* 2006). Nor can the effects of these structural inequalities be explained simply by class mediated variations in individual health promoting or health damaging practices. They operate cumulatively over the whole lifespan, involving complex interactions between the individual and those social and communal supports that maintain health (Blane 2006; DiPrete and Eirich 2006). Such findings are derived principally from studies of morbidity and mortality amongst adults of working age. Secular changes in adult mortality mean that deaths amongst adults of working age are less frequent and are treated as 'premature' and 'preventable'. Making death an event constitutive of old age however leaves open the questions of when death ceases to be 'premature' and what are the true conditions that can be expected in later life. As we have seen there has been a wealth of research indicating universal, secular improvements in late life mortality. Whether this is a result of contemporary social changes or the cumulative effects of processes established at much earlier points in the lifecourse is still hotly debated. In a similar fashion we have seen considerable evidence put forward for declines in morbidity and disability rates. These indicate that many of the predictions made by 'apocalyptic demography' are unlikely to happen. Not only does this suggest that increased longevity will not result in an older and sicker population but that rates of severe disability in later life are actually declining.

As we have seen in relation to the debate around anti-ageing techniques, the steady extension of human life expectancy evident in the twentieth century has led a number of social gerontologists to raise concerns about the collapse of a natural ordering of life (Moody 1995; Vincent 2003a, 2003b). While motivated by what they see as the 'unnatural extension' of later life, facilitated by modern health care interventions, there is agreement that there should be a return to a proper place for an old age that is defined by its connection to death. Most famously, medical ethicist Daniel Callahan (1987) argued that forcing people to live longer than nature decreed would only end in unplanned disaster, individually in terms of prolonged personal suffering and socially in terms of the increased costs of care. In a similar fashion Moody argues that all of the scenarios facing ageing societies, from increasing disability through the compression of morbidity to lifespan extension, lead to a radical displacement of later life. For this reason he suggests, in a quasi-Habermasian fashion, that societies should place voluntary limits on life enhancing treatments after a collectively agreed age in the interests of maintaining intergenerational cohesion. Advocates of this approach imply that there is an exponentially growing personal and social cost arising with each additional year of life won beyond the natural span. What constitutes this natural life span is a point that is never quite settled and this may be deliberate. Callahan implies 75, but is ambiguous. Whatever the actual age chosen, he argues:

> we can have and must have a notion of a 'natural lifespan' that is based on some deeper understanding of human needs and possibilities not on the state of medical technology ... [it is] one in which life's possibilities have on the whole been achieved and after which death may be understood as a sad but nonetheless relatively acceptable event.
>
> (Callahan 1987: 26)

Central to Callahan's argument is that the ideology of 'a natural lifespan' needs to be retained whether or not the actual lifespan is extended beyond that limit. Those cultural values embedded in past notions about the fixed 'structure' or 'stages' of life, he maintains, continue to serve a purpose in today's 'post-modern' world. By offering a socially re-constructed version of a prior foundationalist position concerning the natural limits of human life, Callahan claims a recovered meaning can be established that will help ensure the dignity both of living and dying. A similar approach is offered by Vincent (2003b) who sees that removing the centrality of death to old age has potentially disastrous implications:

> The consequence of this set of beliefs is that science, as culture, misdirects the way in which old age is understood, particularly in the presumption that science potentially can cure death. Rather than valuing life in all its diversity, including its final phase, it leads to the misguided allocation of resources to solving the problem of death. The focus on biological failure sets up a cultural construction of old age which generates and prolongs its low esteem. An irredeemable cultural logic is created: if death is soluble, old age represents a failure. For old age to be its successful conclusion, life requires to be defined culturally not as the continuation of bodily functions but in other ways.
>
> (Vincent 2003b: 682)

This search to 'recover the lifeworld', as Moody (1995) has termed it, where disability and death are no longer equated with failure is doomed to failure. The evidence that the limits of human life are less clear than ever before has become more obvious. What seems most evident is that as more and more people live to be seventy, eighty, ninety and one hundred, the 'nature' of that age becomes open to a wider variety of meanings from which a variety of cultures of ageing can emerge. In some ways the desire to set limits reflects the anxieties raised by the rapidity and openness of contemporary social change. Although collectively agreed limits to the lifespan may not be realisable, less determined social processes may contribute, quite significantly, to the unequal setting of limits. The average circumstances of retired people may be quantitatively better than ever before, but the beneficiaries of these secular trends are to be found disproportionately amongst the wealthy. The length and depth of the third age, such arguments suggest, will be greatest for those who can afford it. If this is indeed the case, it implies very clearly that social factors can and do exercise a continuing influence deep into old age.

Bodily control

In examining the issues of bodily appearance and bodily function we have been examining the social contexts in which ageing embodiment occurs. However, it is the third context of bodily control which gets to the heart of why ageing is not just like other parts of the lifecourse but exists as a submerged threat to agency and identity. Using anti-ageing techniques such as cosmetic surgery to attempt to determine whether and how to 'age' is not just a matter of personal aesthetics. It also represents the massive social dread of old age. While negative attitudes toward old age have been in evidence for centuries (Gilleard 2007) they have rarely played the role that they do in contemporary society. What is unique about the fear of ageing in modernity is that it is represented in numerous cultural and institutional practices that treat 'agedness' as a proxy for decline, neediness and proximity to death (Gilleard 2002). Many writers have seen this cultural attitude as constituting ageism or prejudice to older people, rooted in particular economic and biological power relations (Binstock 1983; Bytheway 1995, 2005). However as the history of old age suggests they are not simply cultural by-products of power relations but they emerge from the processes of bio-ageing itself. McKee (1999) talks of the idea of the 'body drop' as exemplifying this. What he is alluding to is the qualitative shift that occurs when an event such as an older person having a serious fall occurs. Not only are there serious health consequences but there is a realisation that this event marks the crossing of a boundary into a more dependent form of ageing. This is not to downplay the impact of many forms of ageism whether they manifest themselves in the form of institutionalised ageism in healthcare systems, in education, or in the workplace.

Ageism is not just a problem of cultural representation or the lack of respect given to older people. The ageism that takes place in the various institutional practices mentioned above suggests that the solution must lie in the transformation of these social and welfare institutions so that they accord with non-ageist principles. Such an approach fails to engage with the nature of the dilemma that ageing throws up, namely that 'while all would like to live long no one would choose to grow old'. The connection between old age, decline and dependency is ultimately a personal one whether it exists as a reality or as an anticipated fear. Gilleard and Higgs (2000) point out that much of the current discourses around personal ageing are primarily cultures of resistance to age, not ways of embracing old age. These discourses amplify the antipathy to old age that has been present through much of recorded history. In a similar fashion cosmetic surgical practices and anti-ageing techniques are not designed to counteract or to challenge ageism, rather they represent an aesthetic preference not to look like an old person, not to appear elderly. This obviously causes a contradiction between combating ageism and the pursuit of an otherwise disease free 'successful ageing' because if bodily ageing represents an increased risk of developing disability and dying, then all bio-markers of age are associated with such enhanced risks. It is only by not accumulating such markers that an individual can be considered 'successful' in resisting what otherwise seems the destiny of those experiencing longer life spans.

However, the dread of old age is much deeper than just the signs of old age. Andrew Blaikie draws this point out when he writes: 'increased longevity also means more incontinence, more dementia, more bodily betrayals and breakdowns in communication' (Blaikie 1999: 109). While Blaikie may be making a too simple connection between longevity and physical decline he is putting his finger on one of the key issues that situates old age. In a similar fashion, Julia Twigg (2006: 51) points out that the coping strategies of those in 'deep old age' are best seen in terms of a denial of the body or of transcending its limits. Vincent too sees the circumstances of those in residential care as being so stripped of roles and social connections that any expression of identity is severely limited (Vincent 2003a: 129). While these formulations may seem to echo previous approaches to the problem of old age they sit at a very different juncture. The emergence of a third age as an increasingly important arena of choice for older people has thrown into sharp relief those in a fourth age where such choices are absent or severely restricted. Again while writers such as Vincent and Twigg see the fourth age as an unintended consequence of the valorisation of a third age it is difficult to see how the circumstances of those whose bodies have 'betrayed' them can be transformed by purely social means. To a degree those in deep old age are nature's not society's casualties. If death and infirmity in later life are explicable in terms of age alone, the passage through old age cannot be easily represented as the result of personal and/or collective choices in the way that it can be during the third age. The naturalness of disability and dependency in old age suggests a lack of social and/or individual responsibility. The old aged person becomes simply the subject of natural processes while their unrelatedness to the social structuring of the society excludes them from the play of the social. The indeterminacy of class and culture in late old age lead then to the greatest impoverishment of all – exclusion from the processes that establish and give meaning to everyday life. No longer touched by the effects of economic oppression and exploitation, left with a disinvested existence, the very old survive only within the interpretive structures of others – increasingly caught in the webs of significance spun by the functionaries of health and welfare systems.

(Gilleard and Higgs 2000: 162)

We will examine the distinction between the third and the fourth age in a later chapter, but if the fourth age is to be characterised by anything it can be said to be the loss of agency over the body. There are many ways in which loss of bodily control, or the fear of such loss, occur during later life and along with the outward signs of ageing many of these changes are monitored by older individuals. Whilst it would be possible to examine the loss of bodily control in relation to other 'fourth age' phenomena, falls and incontinence for example, none have as much impact in curtailing the potential for ageing individuals to maintain individual identities as cognitive decline. Dementia of whatever description is the progressive loss of both personal and social agency.

The majority of people become resigned to the 'inevitability' of at least some aspects of bodily ageing, but accepting that the mind itself is mortal is more challenging. The irrationality embodied by dementia challenges the idea of the disembodied rational actor that has been so central to modernity. In this sense, senility (to use a pre-modern term) represents the failure of the modern, civilised body. In dementia, the body escapes from its identity as capable of articulating agency. All the behaviours which are associated with 'self care' – looking after oneself, keeping oneself clean, controlling bodily functions and modulating the expression of emotions – controls which Elias (1978) in his history of manners described as central to the civilising process, are eroded in the process of becoming senile.

Shilling (1993) identifies three defining features in Elias' account of the 'civilising process', namely the socialisation, rationalisation and individualisation of the body. Bringing bodily functions increasingly under social control, emphasising the importance of poise and self-control and locating identity specifically within the body represent key historical developments in the emergence of modern ideas about people's relationships with each other and the development of a public and private self. The failure to exercise control – the evident inability to exercise control – effectively excludes the person from participation as an agent within the social world. Dementia is not just a failure of control; it is an unwitting failure of control. It is not the case that the person with dementia has chosen to deviate/transgress or that he or she has been excluded from the civilising processes of society. The progressive loss of choice, of socialised intent is an 'internal' failure and it is this failure that poses such a dilemma for contemporary society.

The term dementia has long been used to express the recognition that some individuals cannot comport themselves in a civilised fashion – and that society is unable to compel them to do so (Berchtold and Cotman 1998). Society rather than the individual, therefore, is supposed to do something about it. However, if the problem of dementia is a problem of loss of self-control and the unwelcome re-emergence of the *uncivilised* body then the failings of the civilised body pose serious problems for the 'post-welfare' state. If dementia is not 'someone's fault', if it is a common and potentially inevitable way in which a large percentage of people will pass their final years – should they live long enough – then the state is faced with either reinstating a 'back to basics' policy of inducing families to care more, or having to plan for those who cannot plan for themselves. The problem is compounded by the emphasis on treating all citizens as customers seeking health and social care services within the framework of contract law rather than universal entitlement.

The vague term dementia has undergone a process whereby it has become synonymous with one condition within it namely Alzheimer's disease. Organisations such as the Alzheimer's Society in the UK represent the carers and sufferers of dementia without seeing the need for more specific categorisation. Gilleard and Higgs (2000) see in this copyrighting of Alzheimer's disease as the real cause of dementia a way of overcoming the dilemmas inherent in dementia by treating the sufferer as a patient legitimately seeking treatment for a disabling neurological condition with laid down protocols and treatment plans. At the conceptual level this approach towards dementia might seem to offer an opportunity of re-civilising senility by allowing it to come under the ambit of bio-medicine. Unfortunately, the aspirations of Alzheimer science have so far outstripped their realisation while it has been the 'carers' who have come to serve as proxy consumers seeking 'treatment' for their partners or parents.

If dementia and its consequences cannot be treated another set of ideas seeks to re-civilise the ageing body under the general rubric of 'discovering the person in dementia' (Downs 1997). Emerging within the health and welfare professions toward the end of the 1980s, this new approach to 're-civilising' the aged body has been described specifically as the 'new culture of dementia care'. According to this approach, the social exclusion of the person with dementia is seen as the consequence of an oppressive and malignant psychology, effectively preventing the person from remaining a member of civilised society (Kitwood 1997; Baldwin and Capstick 2007). In its focus upon the role of a malign social system or structure as the cause of the problems of demented people it shares some of the tenets of both structured dependency theory and the social model of disability. The broad thesis is that 'malignant social psychologies' take away from people 'their last remaining traces of competence and self-respect' leading to a deterioration in 'personhood'. The goal of the 'new culture' is to replace this malignant social psychology with a 'benign' version which 'might over a period even provoke some structural regeneration among the neurones that remain' (Kitwood 1997: 220).

Inevitably responsibility for both the malignant and benign social psychologies lies with other people – families, friends, carers – who are credited with the power/responsibility to re-civilise (Kitwood uses the term 'rement') the dementing person. A small but significant literature has appeared that pursues the process of re-civilising senility by seeking to 'hear the voice of the person with dementia', treating people with dementia as 'users' or 'consumers' of services, seeking out ways of representing their views directly or through the use of advocates (Goldsmith 1996). Attempts to maintain/restore/preserve an identity for the person with dementia involve placing responsibility for his or her continued socialisation in the hands of individual carers. Institutions and institutionalised care are represented as potentially, if not actually, malignant environments responsible in some way for the senility and dementia of those who have been placed there.

The task of these progressive forces is to act as re-interpreters of the language of Alzheimer's. New meanings are attributed to the actions and inaction of the victims of Alzheimer's and a new language taught to carers. Thus equipped with a new map and a new culture, they can discover the person within the disease and rediscover the disease within the person. The rhetoric of this new dementia culture seeks explicitly to re-civilise Alzheimer's. In the process, it seeks radically to alter the culture and civilisation of the broader society which is viewed as giving too much emphasis to 'individuality and autonomy'. By taking reason off its pedestal and re-civilising Alzheimer's, Kitwood claimed a new perspective will emerge that will see: 'a new and vibrant humanism ... gaining ground: more strongly committed, more psychologically aware, more culturally sensitive, more practical and pragmatic than anything that has gone before' (Kitwood 1997: 144).

Such a strategy not only seeks to re-inscribe the person who suffers from dementia but seeks also to re-present the very nature of dementia as part of a much wider and less rational conceptualisation of the individual both as social being and social agent. Gilleard and Higgs (2000: 187) point out that with this move 'The cultural turn it seems comes full circle. Autonomy and rationality themselves need to be re-civilised through a new "Alzheimerisation" of society'.

Alzheimer's disease is probably one of the most widely known medical conditions in the developed world. It continues to inspire a vast research and clinical literature. People of a certain age now joke about developing Alzheimer's when embarrassed by a lapse of memory or attention. Regular Alzheimer's Society 'awareness' weeks ensure that either the subject does not get forgotten or that funds need to be allocated to dealing with it. Although research continues to refer to dementia as a broad umbrella term, studies of dementia and studies of Alzheimer's overlap to such an extent that dementia seems likely soon to be completely subsumed under the term 'Alzheimer's disease and related disorders'. But if Alzheimer's disease is something that provides a name that helps dignify the disabilities of dementia in ways that senility and dementia do not, it is an achievement that comes with a cost. That cost involves pushing dementia into a residual social category of the fourth age, a place where social death precedes biological death. Those excluded from the scientific civilising category of Alzheimer's remain a potential or actual public burden. Other attempts at re-civilising dementia have equally costly consequences. The 'cost' of mental frailty in old age is transformed from a responsibility to be planned for and borne by any 'ageing' state to one that resides primarily with individuals – whether as victims or as carers.

Within societies where lifestyle consumerism and personal recognition play such an important role in the dynamics of everyday life, failure to embody the culture resulting from a loss in the capacity for self-care represents one of the most serious of identity flaws. It particularly challenges the sustainability of any 'culture of ageing'. In debates regarding the limits to human ageing, the mortality of the mind may prove the most important fact in setting those limits. Redistributive policies do not guard against the impoverishment of dementia whilst gender politics address those who care, not those who suffer from dementia. Consumer choice and the technologies of the self seem of little account in preventing the occurrence of dementia or in transforming its meaning. It may be that in the end there is a return of the repressed in that the body determines the final result of the game but this, in and of itself, does not invalidate all the other processes leading up to it.

Conclusion

Faced with the physicality of old age, the changes in appearance and function that are seen socially as defining adult ageing, it seems impossible to argue that ageing can be understood as rooted not in the domain of biology but in social relations. While this view might seem similar to the conclusions drawn by those who seek to re-enchant the lifecourse and reject the significance of the cultural turn in social gerontology, this would be a limited reading of the material that we have presented here. We have outlined three broad topics connected to aspects of the ageing body in order to demonstrate that there is a need to re-focus attention on the contemporary circumstances of ageing rather than view them just through the prism of social policy or social work. We readily acknowledge that the topics that we have chosen have already been the subject of attention by many social gerontologists who have made their own interpretations. Our approach has been to show how areas for gerontological research are not only changing before our eyes but that they need to be understood in very different ways if the study of old age is to maintain its critical function.

6 The birth of a new sociology of health in later life

Introduction

In those western countries experiencing dramatic rises in life expectancy and affluence in the second half of the twentieth century, social understandings and attitudes to the ageing process have undergone profound transformations. These have been at the core of this book so far and need to be at the heart of any reconceptualisation of a sociology of health in later life. In particular there is a need to address the issue of how the relationship between health and ageing changes as ageing also changes. As Kirkwood (1999, 2004) indicates, distinctions between ageing and disease become increasingly blurred and taken for granted understandings of 'natural' ageing are increasingly undermined. Cultural and historical studies have shown how attitudes towards ageing and the old vary across time and cultures (Cliggett 2005; Gullette 2004; Holmes and Holmes 1995). These are important contexts for understanding the ambivalent, sometimes contradictory, responses to the role of medical science in extending the boundaries of longevity and quality of life in old age. As we have seen in previous chapters, naturalistic approaches to ageing tend to view physical and mental decline as a final stage in life prior to death and that this 'natural' process has been distorted by the medicalisation of old age and death (Vincent 2006a). While this has been a familiar refrain since the writings on medicalisation of Ivan Illich (1976) there is the need to make a further distinction between ageing as a norm in the western lifecycle and what is now considered to be 'normal' ageing in these societies. In a similar fashion to the debate on anti-ageing medicine among gerontologists, Rose (2001) emphasises the ways in which new bio-technologies make the boundaries of 'normal' ageing more plastic and open to manipulation. Citing a range of interventions, from hormone replacement therapy to Viagra, he suggests that a 'normal' ageing process is becoming increasingly fragmented by the field of choices made available to those entering later life.

For Rose 'natural' ageing might be seen as a chosen response (from a range of responses on offer) to a stage of life but it is one that exists in a state of growing indeterminacy where the very success of modernist welfare states has led to longevity becoming a normal expectation and life extension something always on the horizon. The consequence of this is that experience of ageing has become increasingly heterogeneous and is accompanied by an increase in uncertainty and insecurity about what later life entails and what constitutes appropriate age related health. Furthermore, the hegemony of social and cultural norms of youth and youthfulness has popularised the ideal of the active pursuit of body maintenance deep into later life (Katz 2005).

This chapter will outline the mainstays of a sociology of health in later life in the twenty-first century. Drawing on the recognition that the separation of old age from the rest of the lifecourse is less and less feasible, the chapter will suggest that as a drawn out period of later life becomes an expectation that most people hold, the effects and dilemmas of ageing reach back further into earlier ages. In order to do this the chapter will address five areas where our understanding and experience of old age are being transformed. First, we consider the rise of the somatic society and the will to health. Second, we consider the impact of the somatic society on what we refer to as the 'Arc of Acquiescence' as individuals anticipate and deal with the impact of age on their bodies. Third, we examine the effect of anti-ageing techniques and medicine on the conventional understanding of the role of health within later life. Fourth, we explore the boundaries between the third and fourth ages, focusing on the way in which these crucial concepts frame later life. Finally, we assess the consequences for later life of the relationship between increased longevity, death and changing attitudes to our own mortality.

The somatic society at later ages

Sociological responses to the advances of molecular biology and genetic medicine can be divided into those who see the geneticisation of society leading to increasing surveillance, control, discrimination and fatalism among the population (Lippman 1992) and those who view these changes as part of a trend towards new and active engagement with the future (Rose 2001). In the former there is a tendency to view human agency as being constrained by advances in new bio-technologies, while in the latter group there is a more optimistic account of human agency where the somatic individual engages in 'novel life strategies' made up of practices of choice, enterprise and self-actualisation. In the Somatic society, personhood becomes reshaped along somatic lines (Novas and Rose 2000). New medical technologies have the potential to re-order life itself leading to the redefining of social and bodily boundaries (Brown and Webster 2004).

One of the areas where these processes are least visible, as far as later life is concerned, is that of the new genetics. This is because genetics is seen by many to be related to the beginnings rather than the ends of life. However, we would argue that as our knowledge of genetics is transformed the effects will increasingly be felt in public attitudes towards what were previously considered to be unavoidable bodily consequences of ageing and in particular the timing of these processes.

As Habermas (2003) points out, advances in bio-sciences have now reached dizzying heights as 'human nature' comes within the remit of bio-technology's intervention and we extend our control over ourselves and our environment (Harvey 1996). The field of bio-technology is one where the speed of change as well as the emergence of new discoveries means that social, philosophical and ethical debates about the consequences of these new discoveries have often found it hard to keep up and are generally reactive rather than proactive. One of the key areas of development in health science is that of preimplantation genetic diagnosis (PGD) that raises the prospect of deliberate and instrumental species change. PGD allows the screening of healthy and unhealthy embryos. Bio-scientists and the large pharmaceutical companies are looking to also breed organ-specific tissue from embryonic stem cells allowing corrections to be made in the genome itself. These advances have meant eugenics is developing in two directions: a negative eugenics based on screening out 'defective' genes and a positive eugenics aimed at enhancing human beings. However, the line between these two different forms is often blurred and the terminology of negative to refer to the selection of undesirable hereditary factors and positive to refer to the optimisation of desirable ones may also be misleading and unhelpful. What is clear is that the combined forces of free markets, neo-liberal social policies and bio-technological progress have meant that it is increasingly difficult to keep a lid on this 'Pandora's box'.

Resistance to these advances (which offer further avenues for controlling nature) are built partly on a sense of our losing control to science (Franklin 2007). Thus attempts at regulation are, to some extent, driven by forces aimed at re-asserting a moralising control. This moralising human nature can appear on the one hand to be both anti-science and against the expansion of freedom and individual autonomy, values that have tended to accompany previous technological developments. But an alternative reading of it is to see it as an 'assertion of ethical self understanding' (Habermas 2003: 25), which is a vital component of our capacity to mutually recognise our autonomy. Seen in this way, instead of being an anti-modern reaction it might be viewed as part of reflexive modernity. With respect to ageing, the advances in PGD offer predictability and control over future potential illness. This suggests that the technology will become one of the key mechanisms by which the effects and dilemmas of ageing reach back further and further into earlier ages.

Rose (2001) argues that the somatic individual accepts personal responsibility for health and is the embodiment of governmentality. Regimes of bio-power define the boundaries to normal ageing and these reject notions of decline and decrepitude. The new technologies of the self are internalised by individuals in a collective 'will to health'. This cuts across the lifecourse, demanding bodily regulation from people of all ages. This view draws heavily on Foucault's (1973, 1977) notion of disciplinary regimes of power and the notion of bio-power (Rabinow 1984). From the late eighteenth century onwards, advances in medical science produced new forms of discipline and control. These ideas became very influential within medical sociology from the 1980s onwards particularly through Armstrong's notion of surveillance medicine (Armstrong 1983, 1995) where the expansion of the medical gaze from individual bodies to populations is highlighted as a key trend in the late twentieth century as was the shift from concerns about disease to a focus on health and risk (Armstrong 2002). Within this paradigm, Public Health policies and health promotion activities are considered to be part of governmentality (Lupton 1995). That is the encouragement of self-regulation through bodily discipline. This has become a key objective of welfare regimes in modern states (Castel 1991; Dean 1999; Foucault 1991).

Drawing on Foucault's work, Katz (1996) identified a discourse of senescence emerging in eighteenth century France capturing the aged body in three interconnected spaces. First, as a system of signification, the appearance of ageing became associated with the symptoms and signs of inner lesions. Second, the aged body became categorised as having a distinct pathology. Third, the aged body became associated with dying. Further applying these ideas to ageing in late modernity, Katz and Marshall (2003) argue that older people are presented with contradictory pressures. The expectation is that they remain active and autonomous, displaying as many characteristics as possible of successful ageing. At the same time the bio-medical and social welfare gaze views their ageing bodies as potentially risky and vulnerable and in need of surveillance and self-discipline. Armstrong (1983) goes so far as to argue that geriatric medicine as a specialty was born directly of the survey and necessitated a continuing intervention whether the patients were in or out of the hospital. While the historical detail may be incorrect with proposals for the establishment of geriatric medicine as a training speciality being proposed independently of such surveys and at earlier points (Warren 1943) the general thrust of his argument is correct with the older patient always being viewed as potentially in need of a health care or social intervention. This sets up tensions between identity and the presentation of self where signs of age-related decline have to be managed so that older people are not completely subsumed under their ascribed status.

The 'arc of acquiescence'

Consumer society rests on an increasing focus on the self as constructed through regimes of the body ranging from plastic surgery and body maintenance to health, fitness and diet regimes. Such regimes, Giddens argues, are geared towards the construction of the 'autotelic self'; a self that embraces and confronts the challenge of risk as a process leading to the positive transformation of the self (Beck 1992; Giddens 1991). Under these conditions of constraint and liberation the body becomes an objectified presence where both health and appearance become sites of new anxieties. These anxieties range from eating the appropriate diet and avoiding the trap of obesity to perfecting the appropriate body shape and having a perfect set of white teeth. The connecting factor between them all is a consumer culture where difference and differentiation not only motivate action but also denote failure. Zygmunt Bauman (1998) relates these ideas to the transformation of modernity from one based around the nation state to one based around consumption. The changes in bodily regime, argues Bauman, mark a move from standardised bodies defined around military and industrial needs to bodies defined by the needs of a consumer society. In a similar fashion to work on governmentality while health concerns become increasingly privatised, welfare systems more and more see their objective as the regulation of populations (Lupton 1995). Differences in forms of bodily maintenance and bodily appearance in this context become key markers of inequality. Just as Bourdieu charted the role of bodily aesthetics as markers of distinction in French society (Bourdieu 1984) Bauman sees bodily regimes and bodily obsession as key markers of an increasingly polarised consumer society. The capacity to resist both the appearance of ageing and bodily decline in later life becomes a form of distinction in itself. When Bourdieu referred to the process of social ageing as 'nothing other than the slow renunciation or disinvestment (socially assisted and encouraged) which leads agents to adjust their aspirations to their objective chances, to espouse their condition, become what they are and make do with what they have' (Bourdieu 1984: 110–11) he was outlining the effect of time and structure on individual trajectories. But in consumer society, despite ample evidence of inequality and restricted social mobility, these trajectories are seen to be matters of individual aspirations and choice. With regard to later life therefore we propose that a useful metaphor for understanding individual and group trajectories of ageing is that of the '*arc of acquiescence*'. This traces the decline associated with a gradual withdrawal from successful body maintenance and the greater acceptance of bodily limits. However, as in most interactions between self and society the curvature of this arc becomes elongated especially among those with the social, cultural and economic capital to support continued engagement with the individualised demands of a somatic society. Just as imperatives to prevent ageing and diseases of old age may colonise discourses of the new bio-technology and so reach back further into early life, so anxieties about regulating ageing bodies may reach forward capturing later life itself in a somatic embrace. For some this manifests itself in doing the daily crossword in order to prevent mental decline, for others it lies in yoga or exercise classes and for others it lies in nutritional supplements or restrictive calorie diets. All of these play roles within the arc of acquiescence. The utility of this concept we would argue is that rather than seeing ageing as a purely personal misfortune or a socially constructed artifice the arc of acquiescence allows for the individual experience of ageing to be situated within a social context all the time being aware that even under the new circumstances of later life issues of capacity and performance are still important.

Anti-ageing medicine and technologies

As we have noted in previous chapters the sociology of the body has not really paid sufficient attention to the ageing body and as a consequence has been unprepared for many of the issues thrown up by anti-ageing medicine and new medical technologies. More familiar with ideas of body modification as transgressive rather than age-related (Pitts 2003) sociologists of the body now find themselves in overlapping positions with social gerontologists who, as we saw earlier, are also grappling with the phenomenon. The rise of the somatic society has focused attention on the ageing body in ways that previously have been seen as the province of gender (Davis 1995). The pressures to extend the arc of acquiescence, based on images of youthfulness and idealised lifestyle are now affecting both genders as the cosmaceutical industry markets greater numbers of anti-ageing products to men as well as women (Dychtwald 1999). These developments particularly affect the middle classes (Featherstone and Hepworth 1991) where the arc of acquiescence is becoming elongated by ever more active and self-conscious attempts to delay the onset of the negative aspects of ageing. Gullette (2004) sees this in terms of cultural life being saturated by the cult of youth but as Elliott (2003) argues these developments are not gender neutral and the objectification of women works alongside the youthful obsessions of consumer society. It is in this space that anti-ageing medicine finds its willing subjects and exerts its influence on the meaning of health.

The rise of anti-ageing medicine reflects the capacity of markets to capitalise on the youth orientation of consumer culture and to promote anti-ageing as a solution to the 'natural' ageing trajectory. The pursuit of desires expressed as new needs is a key part of this in that many anti-ageing treatments can be viewed as being responses to the construction of desires that are doomed to be forever unsatiated. One can become, to borrow a term, age-orexic (D'Souza 2007) and addicted to anti-ageing interventions (Singh and Kelly 2003). Anti-ageing medicine operates at the boundaries of both conventional medicine and bio-gerontology and has been condemned for it (Butler *et al.* 2002). For some, its view of ageing as treatable is a welcome challenge to mainstream gerontology (de Grey 2003; Mykytyn 2006). Obviously, as we have seen, one of the major problems with the term is that it encapsulates such a wide variety of treatments from cosmetic surgery to telomere cellular shortening (Katz, 2005). It is this broadness, we would argue, that makes the area as important for medical sociologists as it is for social gerontologists. Given the rise of new medical technologies, bio-medicine and commercialisation of anti-ageing products the boundaries between medical treatment and beauty treatment become blurred. Bio-gerontological approaches tend to see ageing as a failure to repair defects at the molecular level. In contrast the work of anti-ageing scientists and practitioners seeks to promote the extension of human life span by introducing techniques that prevent many of the conditions that accompany ageing. While bio-gerontologists fight to make a distinction between legitimate attempts to treat old age and the diseases of later life by highlighting the quackery of much anti-ageing the distinctions between the 'cosmetic' and a 'feckless' pursuit of vanity may not be as clear as sometimes presented.

Binstock (2003) highlights the disparaging response to anti-ageing medicine by 51 senior gerontologists who attempted to expose its lack of credentials in a signed document given national prominence in the USA. He analyses this statement as an example of attempts by gerontologists to maintain their own professional legitimacy and their own funding streams. Bio-gerontologists have long opposed what they see as the disproportionate application of research funds to addressing diseases of old age (e.g. Alzheimer's) rather than ageing itself; referring to it as 'Alzheimerisation' of ageing. But more recently their complaint has turned to anti-ageing medicine and the 'hawking' of therapies to what they see as gullible people, through the internet in particular. Binstock cites the position statement on human ageing as an example of boundary work (part of a strategy of professionalisation). To do this he charts the development of research funding for ageing research in the USA. Mainstream gerontology in the USA is funded in excess of $1 billion a year but from the early 1990s onwards its position was being challenged by anti-ageing medicine. He highlights, as key events, the 1994 Dietary Supplement Health Education Act that relaxed the regulation of anti-ageing products leading to a rapid increase in their sales (particularly sales of dietary products). He further cites the setting up of the *Journal of Anti-Ageing Medicine* and Anti-Ageing websites, and in particular the formation of the American Academy of Anti-Aging Medicine (A4M) which has fought battles with the National Institute of Aging over sites of knowledge and the scientific status of anti-ageing medicine. However, the real difference between NIA and A4M may be that the latter believe anti-ageing interventions work at present while the former think they may do so in the future (Moody 2002).

Vincent (2006b) argues that contested scientific discourses on ageing reflect the dominant cultural discourse in the West that denigrates old age and dying. In doing so he identifies four types of anti-ageing science. The first, 'symptom alleviation', is appearance based and can take cosmetic, prophylactic and compensatory forms. This type of anti-ageing is very strongly linked to changing notions of the body and identity. The second, 'life expectancy extension', is disease based and addresses 'diseases of ageing' including cancer and heart disease. The third, 'lifespan extension', is dominated by research at the genetic and molecular level. Here old age is equated with cellular senescence. Finally, 'abolition' refers to the wilder shores of anti-ageing that seek immortality or its equivalent. As we have seen in an earlier chapter there are strong moral judgements associated with the anti-ageing debate and Vincent is explicit in his attempts to bring back notions of a worthy acceptance of biological limits and human finitude. In a similar vein Moody (1995) draws on Habermas to call for resistance to the medicalisation of old age and for a restoration of meaning to old age and death based on communicative rationality and dialogue. The recourse to Habermas should perhaps be expected because it suggests that these developments are being viewed through the prism of ethics rather than in terms of a transformation of the relations of health and healing in modern society (Scambler 2002). In the discussion of anti-ageing medicine we can hear the echo of Ivan Illich's view of medicalisation (Illich 1976) in as much as those who seek out anti-ageing medicine are rendered cultural dupes who, in their desire to access anti-ageing treatments, are fooled by a cult of youth and youthfulness. If people turn towards anti-ageing products and technologies they are viewed as somehow suffering from a form of false consciousness, whereas the adoption of seemingly 'natural' pursuits in later life is valued as appropriate and morally worthy. Clearly technology offers new ways of pushing the boundaries of the human body but as Habermas (2003) argues our response to these challenges should transcend notions of nature versus scientific progress. The ambiguity and complexity that is present within anti-ageing medicine is a useful development in allowing us to see to what extent our views of the relationship between the body and health need to change.

Bauman, in his book *Life in Fragments* (1995), talks about the importance of 'fitness' in contemporary society. However this is not a benign focus on health promotion, rather it marks out one of the chief characteristics of the relationship between the self and society that of constant change and movement. Bodily fitness, for Bauman, is pursued as the supreme goal by many but it is a state that can never be achieved. Instead it:

> lends postmodern culture its unheard-of energy, an inner compulsion to be on the move. It is also a crucial cause, perhaps the prime cause, of its in-built tendency to instant ageing – the neurotic. 'rhyzomic', random, chaotic, confused, compulsive restlessness of postmodern culture with its breathtaking succession of fads and foibles, ephemeric desires, short lived hopes and horrid fears devoured by fears yet more horrid. Postmodern cultural inventiveness may be compared to a pencil with an eraser attached: it wipes out what it writes and thus cannot stop moving over the dazzling blankness of paper.
>
> (Bauman 1995: 119)

Relating this back to ageing it would seem that the technologies that we have been discussing fit very well into this indeterminate notion of fitness and therefore much of the value of investigating how they redefine ageing as well as notions of health is lost if the debate is confined to naturalistic concepts of the body. Rather than pursuing moral arguments about the rights and wrongs of anti-ageing medicine a sociology of health in later life needs to address the lived experience of those who engage, refuse to engage or find themselves unable to engage with anti-ageing practices.

Boundaries between the third and fourth ages

One of the key aspects of the changing nature of ageing is the distinction between the third and fourth ages. While principally conceptual in nature the division between these two categories carries with it very different experiences of ageing (Twigg 2004). It is towards the complex boundary work between the third and fourth ages that we now turn.

The third age

As we have previously noted, Peter Laslett's vision of the third age suggested the emergence of a 'new' period in the lifecourse standing between middle age concerned with the responsibilities of work and child-raising and a fourth age of decline and ultimately death (Laslett 1996 [1989]). Thane (2003) notes that in early modern England there was a notion of a green old age presaging decrepitude that in the twentieth century became known as a distinction between young old age and old old age. This distinction was set out formally by Neugarten (1974) in relation to old age in the American context. Differences between Laslett's conceptualisation of the third age and other European and North American understandings of the term were recognised early on by Laslett. In the second edition of *A Fresh Map of Life* (Laslett 1996) he was particularly critical of attempts such as those by the Carnegie Enquiry (1993, 2000) to define the third age in terms of chronological age. These criticisms have been echoed in a recent attempt by Midwinter (2005) to replace approaches to the third age based on ages or birth dates with a 'stages of life' approach based on the economic status of the citizenry (drawing on engagement in paid work). Midwinter argues that his approach gives a more accurate picture of the relative size of first, second and third ages in the UK over the last 150 years.

These definitional and conceptual differences are important because the term 'third age' has a 'taken for granted' rather than precise meaning. Laslett saw it as a point 'personally chosen' (p. 99) but also as a 'collective circumstance as well as a personal affair'. He therefore saw it as something experienced individually in the context of a society where there is sufficient disposition to act that way. Historically therefore he argued it was a coming together of intellectual, cultural, economic and demographic factors. Because Laslett viewed the third age as representing 'the crown of life' he often over-emphasised its relationship with individual virtuosity. Consequently the distinctions between first, second, third and fourth ages are often blurred. He discusses examples of athletes living both in their third and first ages. He argues that Mozart might be said to have not experienced a second age at all and Jane Austen is described as someone who gave the appearance of living a second age while secretly she was experiencing a third age of masterly achievement. Interesting as these points are they do not really help us distinguish the third and fourth age. Others such as Ball (2002) have tried to think of the third age as comprising six elements all of which represent a 'good life' in old age: family and friends, community service and voluntary work, employment or self-employment, learning and personal development, travel and leisure activities, home and garden. Choosing well for the third age is emphasised here with an almost religious admonition for those who would stray on to the path of dependency:

> The DIY stage of life. The greatest enemy to health, wealth and happiness is dependency; the temptation of dependency is strong for third agers, but needs to be resisted. There will be plenty of time to come to terms with it in the Fourth Age.
>
> (Ball 2002: 4)

In contrast, Christopher King's work draws on Baudrillard's concept of the simulacrum (Baudrillard 1998) to develop a postmodern view of how ageing is portrayed and perceived in an attempt to construct what he terms: 'a "social imaginary" of collective ageing in contemporary consumer society' (King 2003: 156).

As we have seen Gilleard and Higgs (2005) have made the most explicit attempt to theorise the third age by viewing it as a cultural field rather than as representing a 'new' stage of life or a particular social stratum within the aged population. As they write the third age as a cultural field is:

> realised through the activities and discourse of social actors within whose lives it acquires a concrete form. But those forms, those representations of the third age are inevitably ambiguous. It would be a mistake to identify the third age too closely with the characteristics of those in whose lives it is realised. The third age is neither fundamentally gendered, racialised nor reducible to the cultural precipitate of class position or status. It is a cultural field whose boundaries escape the confines of any specific community of interest.
>
> (Gilleard and Higgs 2005: 5)

Taking these issues further Gilleard and Higgs (2007b) argue that what has helped to define this field is the rejection of that which is 'old' precisely because it is old. The generational field that evolved within the lives of the war babies and the baby boomers created a reluctance to identify with that which was 'old' or 'aged'. The third age draws much of its dynamic from this 'generational schism' which was presented publicly and privately as a break with the views and mentalities of an 'older' generation. This resistance to being structured by the social categorisation of old age has become a central habitus of the third age, one that continues to be nourished by ever expanding markets for anti-ageing products and anti-ageing lifestyles.

For Gilleard and Higgs, part of the definition of the third age is its active exclusion of 'old age' and 'agedness'. Consequently it may seem that the fourth age is constructed purely by being not the third age. This seems to be the position adopted by Julia Twigg (2006) who writes that the literature about the fourth age is distanced from the agency of the third age; 'It is about Them not Us. These are the old as constituted in social care' (Twigg 2006: 50). However, Gilleard and Higgs argue against this conclusion. Not participating in the third age does not automatically consign an individual to the fourth age. A key premise of Gilleard and Higgs' argument concerning the third age is that it is a field premised upon the agency of its participants. Not participating in that field is not in and of itself a key attribute of the fourth age. To that extent they claim, the third age has not created the fourth age. Non-participants in the third age may well exercise agency within other domains. Access to the third age and the acquisition of its habitus, varies for historical and socio-structural reasons. The lack of third age habitus does not determine a fourth age identity nor does it instil a 'fourth age habitus'.

The fourth age

It seems clear from this discussion that the fourth age is not simply a life stage development from the third age. While the fourth age has become associated with the dependency and decline of 'very old age' and fourth agers are often identified as the 'oldest old' there is considerable confusion and dispute about definitions of the fourth age which depend on whether it is being approached from demographic, biological, psychological or quality of life perspectives. Certainly attempts to use chronological age as a marker appear too rigid in the face of the considerable variation in the age of onset of the fourth age (Parker and Thorslund 2007). Results from the Berlin ageing study

(BASE) suggest that life in the fourth age is a very negative experience (Baltes and Meyer 1999).[1] The fourth age therefore presents particular difficulties because the oldest old are at the limits of their functional capacity. The pessimistic scenario is that the capacity to intervene successfully in the fourth age is limited with the additional unintended consequence that extending the life span may have the effect of reducing the opportunities of many older people to live and die in dignity.

But this still does not answer the question of precisely how the fourth age is constituted other than through being defined as the physical and mental decline of deep old age. Gilleard and Higgs (2007a) see it as a much more significant category in the articulation of ageing, a category that plays a role for others as much as it defines the predicament of the oldest old. They argue that it is when people are incorporated as third persons in other people's age-based discourse, that they become subjects of a fourth age. This might occur because of a public failure of self-management as much as a specific physiological or psychological symptom. The failure prompts the need to secure the failure by some institutional form of care. Gilleard and Higgs suggest that the failure exists as an '*event horizon*' which once passed allows the older person to become the subject of other 'competent' people's decisions. The use of the event horizon metaphor is designed to indicate that a qualitative break in the older person's competence has occurred and that while it might not be catastrophic it does suggest a point of no return. From this point on the pursuit of agency becomes conditional if not redundant. It is in this way that the fourth age is related to the third age:

> The institutional health and social care practices that have helped demarcate this event horizon, serve as a portal to a more deeply symbolic space that shapes, spurs and renders at times more desperate habitus of the third age. As such, the fourth age acts as a symbolic other, stripped of the social and cultural capital that is most valued, the goods and services, the practices and discourses of choice, autonomy, self expression and pleasure in later life. Looked at through the reflexivity of the third age, it appears as distortions in the mirror, made fathomable by its othering.
>
> (Gilleard and Higgs 2007a: 7–8)

Moreover, unlike the habitus associated with the third age, the fourth age cannot sustain a set of its own dispositions or support forms of symbolic differentiation. Instead, for Gilleard and Higgs, the fourth age acts as a metaphorical 'black hole' of ageing creating fear among those outside its reach, reminding them that deep old age means passing beyond the social world. For observers, influenced in varying degrees by the commodification of consumer society, there appears neither opportunity to articulate a lifestyle within this agency-free environment nor any reason to trust that previous choices will be honoured or acted upon. The fourth age therefore becomes the sum of all the fears lying under the surface of the third age and as such goes further than being a synonym for the oldest old. Likewise in seeing the third age as defined by a cultural rejection of old age we are better placed to see the deeper connections between the somatic society and ageing.

Death and immortality

Our increasing longevity and knowledge of the underlying genetics of disease has stimulated an increasing obsession with the calculability and predictability of disease and ultimately death. So much so that the internet has spawned a number of sites such as 'death clock' and 'death date' that promise to predict our personal demise.[2] Within Public Health, deaths prior to a certain defined cut-off are referred to as avoidable deaths and a good deal of research into the 'old old' is based around predicting functional deterioration and calculating contributions to healthy life expectancy. Bauman (1992) argues that the fact of human mortality and our awareness of it is the basis for social institutions and behavioural patterns that reproduce society. The question we need to ask is what are the consequences for these institutions of mortality becoming increasingly delayed and questioned? Extending healthy life-expectancy and the life span has many profound consequences for human relations including marriage and inter-generational transfers. What does living a healthy active life into one's 90s mean in terms of living in the same marriage? How do inter-generational relationships based on love and reciprocity adjust to both increasing longevity and increasing calculability of life expectancy?

Peter Berger (1967) argued that death was a fundamental feature of all societies and his ideas have been taken up by a number of writers including Giddens (1990) who suggests that the conditions of late modernity have instigated an increase in anxieties about death. These sociological approaches have emphasised the transitions that have occurred in modern society so that death has become less common in infancy and childhood and more associated with later life. Within western culture, death and old age are closely tied in the popular consciousness. As Gullette argues:

> Our metaphors of gravitas – 'weight' of age, 'pull' of death – underlie our associations with 'age'. Ordinary people shake out the death card. Ageing discourse slides into dying discourse without critique
>
> (Gullette 2004: 107)

As we have seen, not only is death associated with old age but also from the mid-twentieth century onwards death became increasingly medicalised (Illich 1976). Sociological studies of the impact of medical science on the experience of death highlighted how the organisation of death in the USA's healthcare system resulted in death becoming routinised and bureaucratised (Sudnow 1967). Other studies showed how hospital staff categorised dying patients at different points along 'dying trajectories' and how this extended clinical control over what is considered a 'good death' (Glaser and Strauss 1968). The sequestration of the dying (Mellor and Shilling 1993) has made it an increasingly lonely, isolated experience (Elias 1985) and the individualised, private and clinically controlled process of dying has become the source of many people's difficulty in coming to terms with their mortality (Mellor 1993).

As outlined in earlier sections of this chapter, advances in medical science and in material affluence have destabilised received wisdom about the biological limits of ageing. Gilleard and Higgs (2000) highlight the blurring of boundaries and the extension of limits through cyber-technology and bio-technologies. These not only offer ways of preventing and delaying the onset of deep old age but also, where the body has entered a phase of decline and dependency, technologies of virtuality offer ways of transcending the biological limits of the ageing body through living/travelling in hyper-reality (Featherstone and Hepworth 1998). These trends have encouraged some to suggest cybernetics break down the boundaries between humans, animals and machines (Haraway 1991). As the limits of physicality are dissolved the positive potentialities of new technologies and genetic modification for post-human life are emphasised (Gane 2006). New medical technologies as Brown and Webster (2004) note are not only delaying death but also redefining the meaning of death. Death and biological finitude no longer correlate as biologically we may continue indefinitely through the immortalisation of cell lines, transplantation, freezing of eggs and sperm and cryonics, etc. At the same time new medical technologies are also being brought to bear on hastening death in ways that allow us choice over the timing and quality of our deaths.

On the face of it therefore the technological advances of second modernity appear to place immortality at the centre of human concerns. Paradoxically Bauman (2001) offers an alternative view suggesting that the imperatives of the consumer society mean that we have entered an entirely new phase where immortality is of no consequence. Instead, it is the throw away, disposable, short-term, impermanence of life that is valued; 'the "long term" is but a package of short-term *Erlebnisse* amenable to endless reshuffling and with no privileged order of succession' (Bauman 2001: 250). Richard Sennett follows a similar argument and uses the metaphor of the ipod shuffle to illustrate the disjointed a-biographical quality of social life in late modernity (Sennett 2006). Does this therefore mean that death has lost its meaning in the same way that ageing seems to have? As Thomas Cole puts it in *The Journey of Life* (1992), if the lifecourse is seen as flexible and fluid does this mean that the finitude of life becomes just another demarcation which should be approached in the same agentic ways as other lifestyle options? This brings us back to the territory of naturalistic views of ageing and death. Should we, as John Vincent (2003a: 159) does, see a good death as not constructed in the right dosage of medication but rather constructed out of 'human relationships and symbols that transcend individuals and their bodies'? Should this be our aim, or are we once again returning to a long departed lifeworld where ageing and death have significance because they are not subject to individual choice? The answers to these questions are maybe not clear-cut but they are nevertheless important and demonstrate once again the fact that many certainties about life and death are not so certain after all.

Conclusion

While it has become commonplace to see old age as no longer constituting a separate phase of the lifecourse this is not the same as arguing that ageing has no impact. Rather as later life becomes more culturally normative and new medical technologies start to affect later life, the effects and dilemmas of ageing reach back further and further to earlier points in the lifecourse. The rise of molecular and genetic science means that we increasingly live in a somatic society where the emphasis is on agentic and reflexive individuals who are able to engage with new genetic technologies in positive ways. At the same time, developments in anti-ageing techniques mesh with a culture of youthfulness and age denial, which throws up many paradoxes for our understanding of the normative in ageing. These changes have led to a greater bifurcation of the boundary between the third and fourth ages while at the same time problematising the boundaries between old age and death. It is by attempting to understand how these aspects of ageing have changed, and how they affect other social institutions and processes, that a sociology of health in later life will prosper.

7 Conclusion

In this book we have addressed the relative lack of attention given to ageing and later life within medical sociology. With respect to research in the fields of health inequality and chronic illness, old age has tended to be marginalised and 'age' has tended to be treated as a controlling variable. Social gerontologists meanwhile have begun to develop frameworks to address inequalities in later life based on concepts such as cumulative advantage and disadvantage, which provide some insights into the processes of stratification and their impact on health outcomes in old age (Dannefer 2003). With respect to chronic illness the focus within gerontology has tended to be on rates of disability and dependency and quality of life in old age (Bond and Corner 2004) perhaps missing some of the insights that have emerged within medical sociology about understandings of and responses to chronic illness. But equally, medical sociology has tended to focus on chronic illness in younger groups at the expense of understanding the changing landscape of health and illness in later life. From within social gerontology itself there is a sense that it has been hampered by its 'interdisciplinarity' and as Phillipson and Baars point out, much research remains 'largely a-theoretical in approach' (Phillipson and Baars 2007: 83). In response to these concerns we outlined the ways in which wide ranging demographic, epidemiological and social changes have transformed the circumstances of, and context to, ageing and in pursuing this we developed an argument for studying later life through the prism of second modernity. We also examined the concerns of social gerontology and considered the extent to which its traditional focus may need to be reviewed in light of wider secular changes and how these particularly affect later life. In the context of the rise of somatic society and second modernity, where individual identities are reflexively and purposefully constructed, we traced research on the sociology of the body and considered different critical approaches within medical sociology and social gerontology to the body in later life. Again we highlighted lacunae with respect to older people and outlined areas where further work needs to be developed. Turning to different approaches within social gerontology towards global change and transitions in welfare provision as applied to later life, we developed arguments that focused on the changing circumstances of ageing and their implication for the construction of individual identities in old age.

In this concluding chapter we return to the arguments relating to second modernity, the reflexive self and old age and outline a prospective research agenda to address the key features of ageing that we have outlined in the main body of the book. In particular, the chapter will discuss the extent to which the main currents in medical sociology and social gerontology have flowed around the ideas of lack and dependency on the one hand and successful ageing on the other. In this sense later life is described in reductionist terms. To avoid being trapped between the construction of welfare failures and the celebratory discourse of a transcendent anti-ageing medicine there is a need for a sociology of later life that is built on the material effects of living later life in late modern societies.

Second modernity and later life

The conditions of second modernity weaken the ties of rationalised institutions and structures and open up new spaces for individuals to purposefully construct self-identity. Although it is important to recognise that there are strong continuities in terms of political, ideological and economic circumstances; considerable changes have occurred in social life over the last 50 years. So much so that Edmunds and Turner (2005) refer to the rise to prominence of a 1960s 'global generation' formed because the traumatic events which helped forge a generational consciousness were for the first time communicated globally and experienced in forms that are disconnected from the boundaries of nation states. They also make an important distinction between events and the representation of events. Because of the rise of a global media, the latter over time, perhaps had a greater influence over the construction of generational consciousness. Events such as the Vietnam war, the rise of protest movements, and new social movements accompanied those features that we have already described such as increasing gender equality, control over fertility, increasing affluence and consumption. All of these led to the freeing up of social attitudes which has had a profound influence over a generation that is now entering later life. However, it is not just positive experiences that should be considered when looking at how later life is marked by discontinuities. In the case of the UK the industrial conflict and inflation of the 1970s had important effects on political attitudes and left deep scars in industrial and working class areas of the country. It is also important to note that many people in retirement today entered mid life during the economic and political changes of the 1980s. Forrest and Leather (1998) for example, argue that the right to buy and early retirement in the 1980 and 1990 recessions are key factors determining the future patterning of retired households. Consequently in the first quarter of the twenty-first century, older home owners will face a varied future in the post-Keynesian welfare state, with some benefiting from these changes and others facing pressure to use their household wealth to meet welfare needs. Older women are twice as likely as older men to be living alone but the trend in solo living is likely to increase in later life as those who contributed to the surge in solo living over the last twenty years now begin to age. Only 4.5 per cent of people aged 65 and over live in communal establishments although this figure rises to over 20 per cent of those aged 85 and over. But older people with limiting long-term illnesses are more likely to live with others and to be in need of formal or informal care (Glaser, Murphy and Grundy 1997). For older people there appear to be two important and connected trends in terms of income and patterns of consumption. In terms of income, older people benefited from the general rise in wealth in the UK over the last 40 years with the proportion of older people in the bottom fifth of the income distribution falling from just under 50 per cent in the 1970s to just over 20 per cent at the beginning of the twenty-first century (DWP 2005). The change in the distribution of income among older households was also significantly affected by a growth in the number of well off retired households who had benefited from generous occupation pensions (Hills 2004). In terms of consumption, levels of expenditure among older households differed considerably from the rest of the population at the beginning of the 1960s but during the last quarter of the twentieth century strong patterns of convergence began to appear both in spending and the ownership of key consumer goods so that by the beginning of the twenty-first century older households might be said to be fully engaged with consumer society (Higgs *et al.* 2007; Jones *et al.* 2008). This has meant that the patterning of consumption has changed with a shift away from necessities (food, clothing, etc.) towards leisure and healthcare items. This rate of change may be different in different countries and the balance of expenditure may also differ with for example the rise in healthcare expenditure being less apparent in the UK and other European countries. In their analysis of 1995 Consumer Expenditure Survey data, Weagley and Huh (2004a) also found that leisure expenditure becomes increasingly important as individuals enter retirement. But income, educational levels and age post-retirement influenced the extent and type of expenditure on leisure (Weagley and Huh 2004b). These examples provide a selective and snapshot picture of some of the social changes that characterised the period in which now ageing cohorts entered adulthood and middle age. While not covering all the events and experiences it should hopefully illustrate that significant social changes occurred that had an impact on a generation in terms of material conditions and political and social attitudes. We suggest that this has to be taken into consideration when examining the rise of a generational habitus that these now ageing groups take with them into old age and that the theoretical framework of second modernity and the reflexive self offers a useful way of gaining a better understanding of social relations and later life in the twenty-first century.

As Giddens and others have argued, a heightened sense of reflexivity becomes the core component of modern identity (Giddens 1991). It is recognised by Giddens that reflexivity has always been a feature of the human condition but in second modernity it develops sharper edges because it saturates the lifeworld as opportunities to self-monitor, reflect and modify individual behaviour have multiplied. In these circumstances, the self becomes a project of identity construction that is increasingly under self-control and autonomy is recognised as both a need and a social expectation. But the 'DIY self' is double edged in that it offers both the freedom to construct individuality alongside the potentially isolating and damaging burden of individual responsibility. Although the postmodern features of this self 'bricolage' have been criticised from a number of perspectives (Savage 2000) it is important to note that Giddens is careful to distinguish between the reflexive self and postmodern notions of the self. The latter is seemingly shattered and dissolved by a fragmented post-modern culture whereas the former concept is based on a knowing and active subject (Giddens 1991). Ulrich Beck (1992) builds on Giddens' notion of reflexivity to describe the construction of individual biographies. Whereas in the past biographies were more socially prescribed and traditionally determined, he suggests that now there is an increasing self-reflexive aspect to the construction of biographies. There are questions however, as to the limits to reflexivity and choice. Adams (2003) for example, argues that reflexivity is a concept that has been constructed around particular values including rationality, instrumentality and calculability and the meaningful 'good' life is founded on notions of a rationally calculating, future oriented, self. Seen in this light, reflexive modernisation is little different from rational choice theory. Indeed in its reification of rational calculating individuals, Adams views it as a cultural construct; a key feature of the normative claims of contemporary culture and asks whether the model of reflexive modernity is little more than the ethnocentric reconstruction of old modernist ideas about the human condition. We would argue that despite this the reflexive self is at the heart of second modernity. The questions that need addressing however are how does the reflexive, knowing, continually contemplative self fit with notions of habitus, routine, unthinking repetitive actions and notions of fate? Giddens (1994) argues that the contemporary world has lost meaning. Tradition had a reinforcing and stabilising effect on memory and on its reconstruction. With the weakening and dissolving of tradition, memory is rendered more problematic and its reconstruction becomes an individual responsibility. The past has lost its grip on us and 'existing habits are a limited guide to action' (Giddens 1994: 92–93). Consequently anxieties about the legitimacy of choices become amplified and there is an increasing reliance on cultural intermediaries who gain social status and cachet through their capacity to remove anxieties from individual choices. While Turner (1995) points out that what he calls the Beck–Giddens approach has very little or nothing to say about the ageing body and the reflexive self we would argue that the concept of second modernity has important consequences for the understanding of ageing. The emphasis both on the autonomous self and the continual construction of the self in relation to a future project leaves individuals in dread of the fourth age and death and the indeterminacy of ageing drives the anxieties and heightened awareness of risk in later life. Later life is also less clearly demarcated from the rest of the lifecourse as previous pathways into post-working life and onwards into old age become more varied. As a result, new aspirations and opportunities are accompanied by new anxieties and concerns. The multiplicity of choices, circumstances and futures for older people raise new challenges for researching later life. For example, gerontological research on retirement transitions has tended to focus on the negative impact of labour market exit and social isolation. However, there is some evidence to suggest that processes of retirement transition involve a complex redefining of a sense of self and identity that need to be understood in terms of individual life histories (Luborsky 1994).

A research programme for later life in second modernity

While the experience of later life has become more heterogeneous it has also become a site of greater social and financial risk (Clark 2003; Minns 2006; Price and Ginn 2006). As the lifecourse becomes more plastic and de-institutionalised, planning for later life is seen to be a key requirement of a 'good citizen' (Giddens 1991, 1998). However, the capacity to engage as a reflexive citizen is context dependent. Research in Canada suggests that such reflexive planning tends to be a feature of high-income groups with a strong future time perspective (Denton *et al.* 2004). If we consider how the notion of retirement as a well defined phase in an institutionalised lifecourse has been eroded, it may be possible to see that structural effects have not disappeared but have taken on new forms. For example, shifts in power relationships in marriage post-retirement have been associated with changes in decision-making powers concerning household consumption. Such shifts are more likely to occur in traditional unequal income relationships as opposed to relationships based on more equal income levels (Webster and Rice 1996). Work by Pahl (2005) suggests that there has been a shift towards more individualised forms of income flows in heterosexual households. This may have benefits for some in terms of decision-making around consumption but there may be unforeseen risks for individualised income and expenditure flows in retirement. Research in the UK suggests that the commonalities of mass fixed aged retirement of earlier periods have been replaced by more individualised experiences of retirement (Vickerstaff and Cox 2005). This fragmentation of experience is however *structured* individualisation because the variety of risks that some individuals may be exposed to in retirement appear to increase without a corresponding increase in the number of choices available. We would argue therefore that second modernity raises new challenges for research addressing later life. In the preceding chapters we have tried to highlight some of these areas and while we cannot claim to cover all the possible areas the following summarise what we believe to be the main challenges:

Second modernity leads to a multiplying of social boundaries and increasing turbulence within and between institutions and individuals Bureaucratic and institutional change may mean that traditional points in the life cycle become more uncertain and subject to plasticity. Points of transition may therefore become increasingly conditional on complex negotiations between bureaucrats and individuals (Heinz 1996). Some suggest that this leads to disjointed status passages (Levy 1996). Institutions are *also* changed by the processes of reflexive modernisation with pressure both to respond to and encourage increased lifecourse flexibility (Settersen 1998). Reflexivity can therefore be seen as a core characteristic of modern institutional and organisational development (Clegg, Courpasson and Phillips 2006). Globalisation and technological change have led to institutions becoming disembedded from their traditional base and this means that they have to be more open to expert and technical modes of thinking. The 'ideal' institutional and organisational forms require openness and flexibility in response to multiple claims to truth. These institutional and organisational forms in turn demand this of the individuals they engage with as those individuals make life choices. According to Giddens this puts projects of self-actualisation on the political agenda because constraints on individual projects are brought to the fore. Gone are certainties about time, nature and bodily boundaries that helped set limits to the self and helped define the self. All boundaries are continually being challenged and redefined. Giddens (1991) also makes great play of the fact that in late modernity 'risk' perception, measurement and anticipation is at the forefront of an individual sense of self. The 'event horizon' that mediates the boundary between the third and fourth ages suggests that a variety of pathways and transitions can come into play in the determining of the ultimate transition. While the move into the fourth age is presaged around decline, loss of function and loss of autonomy, this presents difficulties for welfare institutions as they operate increasingly within frameworks that assume agentic consumer citizens (Gilleard and Higgs 1998). As we noted in earlier chapters it is not a surprise that there is a paucity of sociological studies that interrogate the embodied experience of living in deep old age, however it is more surprising that there are few indeed that examine the boundaries and transitions between the third and the fourth age. With increasing individualisation we anticipate an increase in the points of conflict in the relationships between the public, health and social care systems and older people. In contrast to passive acceptance of levels of service provision, consumer citizens may be

(i)   more likely to pursue claims against and question institutional discretion and rationing

(ii) become more resistant to decisions to move them into the formal categories of the fourth age made by outside parties which reduce their agentic status and

(iii) be vulnerable to exploitation and abuse where their compromised autonomy in the fourth age leads to compromised negotiation in welfare markets.

Second modernity is characterised by a multiplying of rationality with many different claims to knowledge Not only is the experience of ageing increasingly heterogenous but scientific claims about ageing and the treatment of age-related conditions are a highly contested area. As we have seen, battles over the status and legitimacy of 'anti-ageing' medicine are fierce and ongoing. At the same time generations entering later life today were part of new social movements in the 1960s and 1970s and are likely to be more questioning of scientific authority and receptive to different claims to knowledge (Beck 1992). They are also more likely to consider the aesthetic dimensions of ageing embodiment as important criteria in their relationship with healthcare practices. Furthermore, they are likely to be more consumer oriented in terms of their approaches to public and private forms of health provision. These different forces are likely to lead to tensions between scientific, commercial and lay expectations of anti-ageing medicine. Within social gerontology, as we have seen, there is a strong body of thought that views people's use of anti-ageing as a form of 'false consciousness' contrasting this with the morally worthy adoption of seemingly 'natural' pursuits in later life and an acceptance of ageing. Clearly, there are dangers of charlatanism and quackery within anti-ageing medicine but it is also clear that technological advances are extending somatic expectations as well as boundaries. The interest in the participation of older people in high intensity sports such as long-distance running seems a case in point given that it is demanding but still possible. Are these individuals expecting too much and are they acting as irresponsible role models? The distinction between the natural and the artificial seems spurious in circumstances such as these.

Drawing on realist approaches to the body and human nature we have tried to argue that our response to these changes therefore needs to transcend notions of nature versus scientific progress. There are strong tensions between the desires and fears that anti-ageing medicine addresses and the premium placed in society on largely female, youthful bodily forms that drive the growth in markets for anti-ageing techniques. There are also legitimate concerns about the ways in which the expansion of anti-ageing medicines and techniques alongside the pursuit of longevity distorts our priorities in health and may lead ultimately to growing inequalities based on bodily appearance and access to life extending technologies (Vincent 2003a). However, there is ambiguity and complexity in the rise of anti-ageing medicine and this should inform our approach to researching this developing field. Rather than pursuing moral arguments about the rights and wrongs of anti-ageing medicine, a sociology of health in later life needs to address the lived experience of those who engage, refuse to engage or find themselves unable to engage with anti-ageing practices.

Second Modernity is accompanied by increasing individualisation, uncertain careers, unstable lifecourses and new inclusive and exclusive practices creating new forms of inequality. These changes are said to lead to the birth of the 'quasi-subject' where reflexive individuals are expected to choose quickly from uncertain outcomes One of the areas that reflect these uncertainties, instabilities and a multiplication of risks across the life course is that of retirement. The concept of retirement has changed dramatically over the last quarter of a century witnessed by a movement away from fixed and mandatory retirement ages to greater choice, flexibility and insecurity for workers across a range of economic sectors. This trend is likely to continue and will have positive and negative effects captured by a heightened sense of risk associated with retirement decision-making. In the USA, the concept of retirement may be less related to a withdrawal from the labour market and more to a combination of changes in lifestyle or living arrangements with many retirees still participating in the labour market in some way (Wiatrowski 2001). The 'retired' as a group therefore becomes more difficult to define and identify. Rates of early retirement increased significantly from the late 1970s to the early 1990s. This pattern was common to many developed countries. The reasons for and experience of early retirement varied considerably for different groups. Those who were forced into retirement through processes of job shedding often left the labour market at an earlier age, became dependent on the benefits system for income and were less likely to see themselves as retired. In contrast those (either pushed or pulled into early retirement) on higher incomes to begin with were able to retire with generous private/occupational pension provision (Banks and Smith 2006). Analysis of UK data has shown how increasing levels of early retirement were accompanied by greater reliance on means-tested benefits and on employer benefits (Casey 1992). Low wages have been identified as a key common element to a large number of men who took early retirement in the 1980s (Peracchi and Welch 1994). In the USA the impact on income levels of becoming labour market inactive in early later life has been shown to be significant with an average drop in income of 39 per cent with a consequent lower rate of health insurance coverage among this group (Couch 1998). There are marked differences between sub-groups of the early retired and inequalities between those dependent on state benefits and those with other sources of income have increased over time. It is important therefore to examine early retirement in the context of wider secular trends. Loss of job attachment and preference for early retirement may be unrelated to individual personalities, rather they may reflect long-term trends in the economy and labour markets (Ruhm 1995). There is also some evidence to suggest that shifts from Fordist to post-Fordist forms of corporate organisations have had an adverse effect on the career trajectories of older workers with firms tending to place a low value on older workers seeing them as expensive in terms of wage and health insurance costs. Such attitudes appear to cut across sectors of industry with similar trends towards discarding older workers being found in manufacturing and financial services (Quadagno, Hardy and Hazelrigg 2003).

In the UK however, different attitudes towards the older worker have been found in different sectors of the economy, with production and construction sectors making greater use of early retirement schemes and appearing to lag behind other sectors such as service and finance in terms of strategies to address older workers (Taylor and Walker 1994). Pressures to shed or retain older workers wax and wane with economic cycles. With the pressure of an ageing population on welfare and pension systems, governments are now keen to promote strategies to encourage workers to stay in their jobs. Overall income levels in later life increased during the last quarter of the twentieth century. In the USA, for example, between 1969 and 1992 wealth from employer provided pensions increased by 150 per cent in real terms. However, this growth was also accompanied by increasing inequality in the distribution of wealth among older people (Gustman and Steinmeier 2000). In later life the relationship between age and wealth over the lifecycle has been shown to be context dependent with high social status appearing to delay the age at which post-retirement falls in wealth commence (Land and Russell 1996). Furthermore, analysis of income dynamics over the lifecycle has shown that while income trajectories are influenced by the experience of life events at particular stages of the lifecycle there is considerable heterogeneity in income trajectories following different life events (Rigg and Sefton 2006). Analyses of Italian household income data suggests that the lifecycle effects are modified by other factors so that although there is a general decline in income and wealth in later life there is considerable population heterogeneity in the experience of reductions in wealth with rates being considerably lower for richer households and high education households (Jappelli 1999). The trends in life expectancy, better health in later life and early retirement pose particular challenges for welfare systems. Comparative research in this area is still underdeveloped but studies indicate that differences in labour market conditions across space and time coupled with differences in welfare support levels have an impact on the experience of retirement in different countries. For example a comparative analysis of UK and German data indicates that income mobility in old age is more pronounced in the UK and that in both countries downward income mobility in retirement was associated with widowhood, earlier bouts of unemployment and changes in living arrangements (Zaidi, Frick and Buchel 2005).

Levels of income in retirement also display a very strong gender effect. As Ginn and Arber (Ginn 2003; Ginn and Arber 1995) have shown that the gendered division of domestic work and responsibility has a profound impact on the type of employment women are able to undertake and consequently their membership of and contribution to occupational pension schemes. Women are at greater risk of experiencing poverty in later life and this is related both to their capacity to generate individual adequate pension provision over the lifetime of their engagement with the labour market and to the risk of dependence on the pensions of male partners. Women are particularly vulnerable to the detrimental impact on pension income of divorce and recent evidence suggests that this may have a strong cohort effect with younger women being at particular risk (Shuey and O'Rand 2006). The health effects of both anticipating retirement and retirement itself are complex. Research in this area has been influenced considerably by the cumulative deprivation model that has underpinned evidence of inequalities in health outcomes in middle age being influenced by the accumulated deprivation at earlier stages of the lifecourse. However, evidence for the capacity of the model to explain patterns of health in later life is weak. Indeed, a study of mortality among older inhabitants of Oslo found no clear evidence of a cumulative effect of deprivation instead finding social conditions in later life itself being the important factor in risk of mortality (Naess, Hernes and Blane 2006). It is important however, to recognise that the impact of labour market changes in the 1980s may have an effect on the experience of retirement for cohorts who entered retirement at that time as well as cohorts entering retirement subsequent to these changes. Secondary analysis of UK data from the 1980s and 1990s indicates that early exit from the labour market is accompanied by falls in levels of self-reported well-being and that there are inequalities in ageing processes that are strongly related to the experience of deprivation at the time of labour market exit/retirement (Bellaby 2006). Early labour market exit into unemployment or early retirement has been found to impact negatively on mortality rates. An important feature of this trend is that it persists after controlling for other variables such as socio-economic condition, health behaviour and other health indicators suggesting a causal effect, though the effect may be non-specific in that an increased risk of death has been found in relation to cancer and cardiovascular disease (Morris, Cook and Shaper 1994). It is difficult to untangle the effects of prior illness and selection on rates of mortality in retirement. However, some studies suggest that once retirement for disability reasons is controlled for there is a still an adverse effect on health/mortality of retirement itself (Quaade *et al.* 2002). A follow up study of workers in the US petroleum and petrochemical industry found that retiring early was not associated with better survival and workers who retired at 55 had higher mortality rates than workers who remained in work up to age 65 (Tsai *et al.* 2005). For retirement therefore, there seems to be a need to undertake further research addressing the impact of unstable careers and lifecourse risks on outcomes in later life and the presence of ageing cohorts in large longitudinal surveys will make this increasingly possible.

Second modernity is an increasingly insecure social order where individuals become authors of their own biographies and construct narratives that imbue the prevailing uncertainties with meaning The 'self-reflexive' individual faces an open future with multiple possibilities. In this context facing up to risks is based on the purposeful setting of goals connected to the past and guided by a need for authenticity. But what does this mean for older people? The danger of valorising the ideal of the quasi-subject is that in its orientation towards the future it leaves older people behind. As people live longer and healthier lives their sense of the future will also change. But the emphasis on the reflexive self only has meaning as long as there is a future trajectory and expectation – a purpose in life. The norm of reflexivity may be accompanied by a heightened fear and dread of ageing, bodily decline and death. In second modernity where the emphasis is on individualisation and risk, individual trajectories in later life no longer follow predetermined paths of renunciation and adjustment. Increasingly these trajectories are expected to be matters related to individual aspirations and choice. In this book we have proposed a useful metaphor for understanding individual and group trajectories of ageing, that of the *arc of acquiescence*. This traces the decline associated with a gradual withdrawal from bodily maintenance and acceptance of bodily limits. However, within the context of late modernity the curvature of this arc becomes elongated particularly among those with the social, cultural and economic capital to support continued engagement with the individualised demands of a somatic society. Consequently anxieties about regulating ageing bodies may capture later life itself in a somatic embrace. As we have seen in earlier chapters the conditions of late modernity have instigated an increase in anxieties about death. Death has become less common in infancy and childhood and more associated with later life and for some theorists the technological advances of late modernity place immortality at the centre of human concerns. Drawing on the work of Bauman (2001) and Sennett (2006) we have attempted to look at how the rise of consumer society affects these concerns. The disjointed biographical features of life in second modernity may lead to conflicts and contradictions in later life. So the shifting boundaries between old age and death also appear to be spaces where we are witnessing the rise of new conflicts of class and social location based around individual capacities to engage with new technological advancements and the privatised nature of dying. It is in these spaces that we suggest medical sociology needs to develop new research agendas.

Finally we need to be aware, as Bryan Turner (2004) reminds us, that any sociological analysis needs to involve an historical analysis of the conditions under which the human body is represented. The changing relationship between self and society has undergone profound changes and we have attempted to incorporate this by using the idea of 'generational habitus' which as we have pointed out has particular salience in relation to the articulation of the third age. However, Turner takes these thoughts further by pointing out that the collective memory of ageing has a powerful effect not only in terms of personal memories and nostalgia but also in relation to representations of youth and we would argue later life. Part of the generational view of what ageing means could be bound up in collective memories of how it seemed to be for the cohorts that went before them and it could be this memory that influences their attitudes towards old age. Again, with the decline of an overarching institutionalised lifecourse it may be that fictive elements become more important than in the past and this suggests another potential research avenue.

Conclusion

It is possible to view the individualisation of consumer society in positive and negative terms. For example, Elliott and Lemert (2006) draw on the theories of Giddens, Beck and others to argue that individuals respond to the stresses and turbulences of globalisation by 'remaking themselves from the inside'. There is an element of compulsion here in that individuals are required and expected to be active, engaged and purposeful actors in their own biographies. It is not surprising that some interpret this as a form of 'manipulated individualisation' that invades the life world by means of mechanisms of exploitation and accumulation. However, this perspective perhaps overly emphasises the 'passiveness' of individuals in the face of global forces. A more moralistic take on individualism, which Elliot and Lemert refer to as 'isolated privatism', suggests that the self has lost its moral core with society being increasingly made up of shallow and empty individuals obsessed with the surface impressions of their own lives. While resonating with much criticism of postmodern consumer culture and its obsession with celebrity and youth these perspectives also seem simplistic in the way they appear to assume that individuals are incapable of both individualism and purposively communitarian activity in the public sphere. Finally, reflexive individualism, they argue, refers to the self facing up to heightened conditions of risk in second modernity. Modern society is increasingly detraditionalised and requires of individuals a concomitant increase in emotional literacy and cosmopolitanism. This does not necessarily require a capitulation to the individualising, privatising and isolating forces of world capitalism. There are countervailing forces of community, solidarity and cooperation that can still be drawn upon but in new contexts and new guises.

In this book we have tried to offer a counterbalance to the (i) lack of attention given within medical sociology to later life and (ii) the tendency within social gerontology to focus on dependency, viewing older adults as structurally defined. In second modernity the self must strive for authenticity – but whether this authenticity is connected to high or low culture or particular moral values should be left open. These imperatives open up new possibilities for later life when they coincide with access to forms of social, cultural and economic capital. But where such forms are limited, where autonomy is compromised and the self is dissolving, the same imperatives potentially construct a very cold, hazardous and unwelcome later life. It is our view that it is in the difficult, often uncomfortable, spaces between these possibilities that we may find ways of constructing a sociology of health in later life.

We began this book by quoting Tom Kirkwood the eminent biogerontologist and it seems appropriate that we leave the last words to him:

> The freedom to make – and continue making – choices is probably the greatest single index of well-being. Choice matters in ageing

for two very powerful reasons. First, although many of the fruits of the scientific lie in the future, scientific understanding of the ageing process already tells us that there is a great deal that we can do right now by making the right choices. Second, as we get older, choice often seems to be taken away. The infirmity of age undoubtedly sets barriers to certain kinds of choice, while financial hardship – an all too common companion of old age – sets others. But choice tends to be limited by age much more than is really necessary, through either negative expectations or just poor planning. The revolution in longevity puts choice high on the list of priorities.

(Kirkwood 2001: 47–48)

Notes

4 New developments in social gerontology

1 The terms de-commodification and re-commodification are drawn from the work of Esping-Andersen in his seminal work *The Three Worlds of Welfare Capitalism* (1990) where he points out that one of the functions of welfare policy has been to allow sections of the population to have an income and resources not dependent on their place in the labour market. State retirement pensions took older people out of the labour market by giving them a replacement income thus de-commodifying their position in society. The marketisation of many pension schemes has not only created greater inequality in later life but has also re-commodified the relationship that retirees have with the market. Similar processes of re-commodification can also be seen within health and social care policy with marketisation and the introduction of the cash nexus into individualised service delivery.

6 The birth of a new sociology of health in later life

1 In their review of research on the oldest old (Baltes and Smith 2003) suggest that the fourth age entails a level of vulnerability and unpredictability that is distinct from the positive views of the third age. The Berlin ageing study (BASE) which conducted a series of investigations looking at ageing between the ages of 70 and 100 came to similar conclusions (Baltes and Mayer 1999). Smith and Baltes (1999) argue that subjective well-being follows a negative pathway after 80 and that there is heterogeneity of functioning against an average decline in levels of cognitive ability. Furthermore, when compared to the third age, the fourth age is associated with increased risk of poor psychological profiles and these profiles in the fourth age are death related (i.e. predictive of death). If this wasn't bad enough Smith (2001) argues that cumulative health-related chronic life strains in the fourth age constrain older people's capacity to have a positive sense of well-being.

What is not resolved by these kinds of studies however is whether there is age-related change in the fourth age that is independent of death-related change. Some refer to the paradox of stability in subjective well-being in the fourth age versus multiple psycho-social decline and increasing health morbidity at the same ages as a paradox. This paradox may be related to people's capacity to adapt to worsening conditions (Baltes and Mayer 1999). Schilling (2005) however, relates life satisfaction to cohort effects and an acceleration of age-related decline in the old old.

2 The Death Clock (2007) describes itself as 'The Internet's friendly reminder that life is slipping away' and invites individuals to enter basic demographic details so that they can be provided with the predicted date of their death and a countdown to that date in seconds.

References

Aaron, H. Shoven, J., and Friedman, B. (1999) *Should the United States Privatize Social Security?* Cambridge MA: MIT Press.

Abbas, A. (2004) The embodiment of class, gender and age through leisure: a realist analysis of long distance running, *Leisure Studies*, 23 (2): 159–75.

Achenbaum, W. (1978) *Old Age in a New Land: The American Experience since 1790*, Baltimore: Johns Hopkins University Press.

—— (1995) *Crossing Frontiers: Gerontology Emerges as a Science*, Cambridge: Cambridge University Press.

Adams, M. (2003) The reflexive self and culture: a critique, *British Journal of Sociology*, 54 (2): 221–38.

Annandale, E. (1998) *The Sociology of Health and Medicine: A critical introduction*, Cambridge: Polity Press.

Annandale, E. and Hunt, K. (Eds.) (2000) *Gender Inequalities and Health*, Buckingham: Open University Press.

Arber, S. (1994) Gender health and ageing, *Medical Sociology News*, 20: 14–22.

—— (2006) Gender trajectories: how age and marital status influence patterns of gender inequality in later life, in S.O. Daatland and S. Biggs (Eds.) *Ageing and Diversity, Multiple Pathways and Cultural Migrations*, 61–78, Bristol: Policy Press.

Arber, S. and Ginn, J. (1993) Gender and inequalities in health in later life, *Social Science and Medicine*, 36: 33–46.

—— (1995) *Connecting Gender and Ageing: A Sociological Approach*, Milton Keynes: Open University Press.

Arber, S. and Lahelma, E. (1993) Inequalities in womens and mens ill-health – Britain and Finland compared, *Social Science and Medicine*, 37 (8): 1055–68.

Armstrong, D. (1983) *Political Anatomy of the Body: Medical Knowledge in Britain in the Twentieth Century*, Cambridge: Cambridge University Press.

—— (1995) The rise of Surveillance Medicine, *Sociology of Health and Illness*, 17: 393–404.

—— (2002) *A New History of Identity, a Sociology of Medical Knowledge*, Basingstoke: Palgrave.

Attanasio, O.P. and Emmerson, C. (2003) Mortality, Health Status, and Wealth, *Journal of the European Economic Association*, 1 (4): 821–50.

Baars, J. (1991) The challenge of critical gerontology: The problem of social constitution, *Journal of Ageing Studies*, 5 (3): 219–43.

Baars, J., Dannefer, D., Phillipson, C. and Walker, A. (Eds.) (2006) *Aging, Globalization and Inequality: The New Critical Gerontology*, Amityville, NY: Baywood Publishing.

Baldwin, C. and Capstick, A. (Eds.) (2007) *Tom Kitwood on Dementia: A Reader and Critical Commentary*, Maidenhead: Open University Press.

Ball, C. (2002) Reflections on the Third Age, *Quality in Ageing – Policy, practice and research*, 3 (2): 3–5.

Ballard, K., Kuh, D. and Wadsworth, M. (2001) The role of the menopause in women's experiences of the 'change of life', *Sociology of Health and Illness*, 23: 397–424.

Baltes, P.B. and Mayer, K.U. (Eds.) (1999) *The Berlin Ageing Study: Ageing form 70 to 100*, Cambridge: Cambridge University Press.

Baltes, P.B. and Smith, J. (2003) New frontiers in the future of aging: From successful aging of the young old to the dilemmas of the fourth age, *Gerontology*, 49 (2): 123–35.

Banks, J. and Smith, S. (2006) Retirement in the UK, *Oxford Review of Economic Policy*, 22 (1): 40–56.

Bardasi, E., Jenkins, S. and Rigg, J. (2002) Retirement and the income of older people: a British perspective, *Ageing and Society*, 22: 131–59.

Barnes, C., Mercer, G. and Shakespeare, T. (1999) *Exploring Disability, A Sociological Introduction*, Cambridge: Polity Press.

Barton, A. and Mulley, G. (2003) History of the development of geriatric medicine in the UK, *Postgraduate Medical Journal*, 79 (930): 229–34.

Bass, S. (2006) The need for theory: Critical approaches to social gerontology, *Gerontologist*, 46 (1): 139–44.

Baudrillard, J. (1993) *Symbolic Exchange and Death*, London: Sage.

—— (1998) *The Consumer Society*, London: Sage.

Bauman, Z. (1992) *Mortality, Immortality and Other Life Strategies*, Cambridge, Polity Press.

—— (1995) *Life in Fragments*, Cambridge: Polity.

—— (1998) *Globalisation*, Cambridge: Polity.

—— (1998) *Work, Consumerism and the New Poor*, Buckingham: Open University Press.

—— (2000) *Liquid Modernity*, Cambridge: Polity.

—— (2001) *The Individualized Society*, Cambridge: Polity.

—— (2004) *Identity*, Cambridge: Polity.

Beck, U. (1992) *Risk Society, Towards a New Modernity*, London: Sage.

—— (2000) *The Brave New World of Work*, Cambridge: Polity.

—— (2005) *Power in the Global Age*, Cambridge: Polity.

—— (2006) *The Cosmopolitan Vision*, Cambridge: Polity Press.

Beck, U. and Sznaider, N. (2006) Unpacking cosmopolitanism for the social sciences: a research agenda, *The British Journal of Sociology*, 57 (1): 1–23.

Beck, U., Bonss, W. and Lau, C. (2003) The theory of reflexive modernization, problematic, hypotheses and research programme, *Theory, Culture and Society*, 20 (2): 1–33.

Beck, U., Giddens, A. and Lash, S. (1994) *Reflexive Modernization: Politics, Tradition and Aesthetics in the Modern Social Order*, Oxford: Blackwell.

Beckett, M. (2000) Converging health inequalities in later life – an artefact of mortality selection? *Journal of Health and Social Behaviour*, 41: 106–9.

Beck-Gernsheim, E. (2002) *Reinventing the Family: In Search of New Lifestyles*, Cambridge: Polity.

Bell, S. (1992) Political gynecology: gynecological imperialism and the politics of self-help, in P. Brown (Ed.) *Perspectives in Medical Sociology*, Ill: Waveland Press.

Bellaby, P. (2006) Can they carry on working? Later retirement, health, and social inequality in an aging population, *International Journal of Health Services*, 36 (1): 1–23.

Berchtold, N. and Cotman, C. (1998) Evolution in the conceptualization of dementia and Alzheimer's disease: Greco-Roman period to the 1960s, *Neurobiology of Aging*, 19: 173–89.

Berger, P. (1967) *Sacred Canopy*, New York: Anchor.

Best, S. (2007) The social construction of pain: an evaluation, *Disability and Society*, 22 (2): 161–71.

Beynon, H. (1999) A classless society? in H. Beynon. and P. Glavanis (Eds.) *Patterns of Social Inequality*, London: Longman.

Biggs, S. (1999) *The Mature Imagination*, Buckingham: Open University Press.

—— (2004) Age, gender, narratives and masquerades, *Journal of Aging Studies*, 18: 45–58.

Binstock, R.H. (1983) The aged as scapegoat, *Gerontologist*, 23: 136–43.

—— (2003) The war on 'anti-aging medicine', *Gerontologist*, 43 (1): 4–14.

—— (2004) anti-aging medicine: The history, anti-aging medicine and research: A realm of conflict and profound societal implications, *Journals of Gerontology Series A: Biological Sciences and Medical Sciences*, 59: B523–B533.

Blackburn, R. (2002) *Banking on Death or, Investing in Life: The History and Future of Pensions*, London: Verso.

Blaikie, A. (1999) Can there be a cultural sociology of ageing? *Education and Ageing*, 14 (2): 127–39.

—— (2006) Vision of later life: Golden cohort to Generations Z, in J.A. Vincent, C.R. Phillipson and M. Downs (Eds.) *The Futures of Old Age*, 12–19, London: Sage.

Blane, D. (1996) Collecting retrospective data: development of a reliable method and a pilot study of its use, *Social Science and Medicine*, 42: 751–57.

—— (2006) Commentary: the place in life course research of validated measures of socioeconomic position, *International Journal of Epidemiology*, 35: 139–140.

Blane, D., Netuveli, G. and Bartley, M. (2007) Does quality of life at older ages vary with socio-economic position? *Sociology*, 41: 717–726.

Blaxter, M. (2000) Class, time and biography, in S. Williams, J. Gabe and M. Calnan (Eds.) *Health, Medicine and Society Key Theories and Future Agendas*, London: Routledge.

Bloom, S.W. (2002) *The Word as Scalpel, a History of Medical Sociology*, Oxford: Oxford University Press.

Bond, J. and Corner, L. (2004) *Quality of Life and Older People*, Buckingham: Open University Press.

Bourdieu, P. (1984) *Distinction: A Social Critique of the Judgement of Taste*, London: Routledge.

Bowling, A. (2007) Aspirations for older age in the 21st century: What is successful aging? *International Journal of Aging and Human Development*, 64 (3): 263–97.

Bradley, H. (1996) *Fractured Identities: Changing Patterns of Inequality*, Cambridge, Polity.

Breeze, E., Jones, D.A., Wilkinson, P., Bulpitt, C.J., Grundy, C. and Latif, A.M. (2005) Area deprivation, social class, and quality of life among people aged 75 years and over in Britain, *International Journal of Epidemiology*, 34 (2): 276–83.

Brook, D. (1998) Enhancement of human function: some distinctions for policymakers, in E. Parens (Ed), *Enhancing Human Traits: Ethical and Social Issues*, Washington: Georgetown University Press.

Brown, N. and Webster, A. (2004) *New Medical Technologies and Society: Reordering Life*, Cambridge: Polity Press.

Bullington, J. (2006) Body and self: a phenomenological study on the ageing body and identity, *Journal of Medical Ethics and Medical Humanities; medical humanities*, 32: 25–31.

Burgess, E. (1960) *Aging in Western Societies*, Chicago: Chicago University Press

Burkitt, I. (1999) *Bodies of Thought: Embodiment, Identity and Modernity*, London: Sage.

Burr, J.A., Caro, F.G. and Moorhead, J. (2002) Productive aging and civic participation, *Journal of Aging Studies*, 16: 87–105.

Bury, M. (1982) Chronic illness as biographical disruption, *Sociology of Health and Illness*, 8 (2): 137–69.

—— (2000) Health ageing and the life course, in S.J. Williams, J. Gabe and M. Calnan (Eds.) *Health, Medicine and Society, Key Theories, Future Agendas*, 87–106, London: Routledge.

Bury, M. and Gabe, J. (2004) *The Sociology of Health and Illness: A Reader* London: Routledge.

Butler, R., (2002) The study of productive aging, *Journals of Gerontology B Psychological Sciences and Social Sciences*, 57: 323.

Butler, R., Fossel, M., Harman, S., Heward, C., Olshansky, S., Perls, T., Rothman, D., Rothman, S., Warner, H., West, M. and Wright, W. (2002) Is there an anti-aging medicine? *Journals of Gerontology A: Biological and Medical Sciences*, 57: 333–38.

Bytheway, B. (2005) Ageism and age categorization, *Journal of Social Issues*, 61: 361–74.

—— (1995) *Ageism*, Milton Keynes: Open University Press.

Bytheway, B. and Johnson, J. (1998) The sight of age, in S. Nettleton, and J. Watson (Eds.) *The Body in Everyday Life*, 243–57, London: Routledge.

Calasanti, T.M. (1999) Feminism and gerontology: Not just for women, *Hallym International Journal of Aging*, 1: 44–55.

—— (2004) New directions in feminist gerontology: An introduction, *Journal of Aging Studies*, 18: 1–8.

Calasanti, T.M. and Zajicek, A.M. (1993) A socialist-feminist approach to aging: embracing diversity, *Journal of Aging Studies*, 7 (2): 117–31.

Callahan, D. (1987) *Setting Limits: Medical Goals in an Aging Society*, New York: Simon and Schuster.

Carnegie Enquiry (1993) *Life, Work and Livelihood in the Third Age*, Carnegie UK Trust.

—— (2000) *A Decade of Progress and Change, A report on Ten Years' Activity and Action on the Third Age*, Carnegie UK Trust.

Casey, B. (1992) Paying for early retirement, *Journal of Social Policy*, 21: 303–23.

Castel, R. (1991) From dangerousness to risk, in Burchell, G., Gordon, C. and Miller, P. (Eds.) *The Foucault Effect: Studies in Governmentality*, 281–98, London: Harvester Wheatsheaf.

Castles, F.G. (2002) The future of the welfare state: Crisis myths and crisis realities, *International Journal of Health Services*, 32 (2): 255–77.

Chamberlayne, P., Bornat, J. and Wengraf, T. (2000) (Eds.) *The Turn to Biographical Methods in Social Science*, London: Routledge.

Cichon, M. (2004) *Approaching a Common Denominator? An Interim Assessment of World Bank and ILO Positions on Pensions*, Geneva: ILO.

Clark, G. (2003) Pension security in the global economy: Markets and national institutions in the 21st century, *Environment and Planning A*, 35: 1339–56.

Clarke, J., Smith, N. and Vidler, E. (2005) Consumerism and the reform of public services: inequalities and instabilities, in M. Powell, L. Bauld and K. Clarke (Eds.) *Social Policy Review*, 17: 167–82.

Clegg, S., Courpasson, D. and Phillips, N. (2006) *Power and Organizations*, London: Sage.

Cliggett, L. (2005) *Grains from Grass: Aging, Gender and Famine in Rural Africa*, Ithaca: Cornell University Press.

Cockerham, W.C., Rütten, A. and Abel, T. (1997) Conceptualising contemporary health lifestyles: moving beyond Weber, *The Sociological Quarterly*, 38 (2): 321–342.

Cole, T. (1992) *The Journey of Life: A Cultural History of Aging in America*, Cambridge: Cambridge University Press.

Collier, A. (2003) *In Defence of Objectivity*, London: Routledge.

Conway, S. and Hockey, J. (1998) Resisting the 'mask' of old age?: the social meaning of lay health beliefs in later life, *Ageing and Society*, 18: 469–94.

Couch, K.A. (1998) Late life job displacement, *Gerontologist*, 38 (1): 7–17.

Crimmins, E.M. (2004) Trends in the health of the elderly. *Annual Review of Public Health*, 25: 79–98.

Crompton, R. and Lyonette, C. (2005) The new gendered essentialism – domestic and family choices and their relation to attitudes, *British Journal of Sociology*, 56: 601–20.

Crossley, N. (2001) *The Social Body: Habit, Identity and Desire*, London: Sage.

Cruikshank, M. (2003) *Learning to be Old: Gender, Culture and Aging*, Lanham: Maryland: Rowman and Littlefield.

Cumming, E. and Henry, W. (1961) *Growing Old: The Process of Disengagement*, New York: Basic Books.

D'Souza, C. (2007) My name is Christa. I'm an age-orexic, *Observer Woman*, May 2007: 21–25.

Dannefer, D. (2003) Cumulative advantage/disadvantage and the life course: cross-fertilizing age and social science theory, *Journals of Gerontology*, 58B (6): S327–37.

Davies, S. (2004) Reflexive planning for later life, *Canadian Journal on Aging-Revue Canadienne du Vieillissement*, 23: S71–S82.

Davis, K. (1995) *Reshaping the Female Body: The Dilemma of Cosmetic Surgery* New York: Routledge.

de Beauvoir, S. (1993) [1949] *The Second Sex*, London: Everyman's Library.

de Grey, A. (2003) The foreseeability of real anti-aging medicine: focusing the debate, *Experimental Gerontology*, 38: 927–34.

—— (2007) *Ending Ageing*, New York: St. Martin's Press.

Dean, M. (1999) *Governmentality: Power and Rule in Modern Society*, London: Sage.

Deleuze, G. and Guattari, F. (1988) *A Thousand Plateaus: Capitalism and Schizophrenia*, London: Athlone Press.

Denton, M. (2007) The gender wealth gap: Structural and material constraints and implications for later life, *Journal of Women and Aging*, 19 (3/4).

Denton, M.A., Kemp, C.L., French, S., Gafni, A., Joshi, A., Rosenthal, C.J. and Davies, S. (2004) Reflexive planning for later life, *Canadian Journal on Aging*, 23, (Supplement 1): S71–S82.

Denton, M.A., Kemp, C.L., French, S., Gafni, A., Joshi, A., Rosenthal, C.J., and Department of Work and Pensions (2005) *Focus on Older People*, HMSO: Newport.

DiPrete, T.A. and Eirich, G.M. (2006) Cumulative advantage as a mechanism for inequality: a review of theoretical and empirical developments, *Annual Review of Sociology*, 32: 271–97.

Donkin, A., Goldblatt, P. and Lynch, P. (2002) Inequalities in life expectancy by social class, 1972–99, *Health Statistics Quarterly*, 15: 5–15.

Downs, M. (1997) The emergence of the person in dementia research, *Ageing and Society*, 17: 597–608.

DWP Department of Work and Pensions (2005) *Focus on Older People*, London: HMSO.

Dychtwald, K. (1999) *Age Power: How the 21st Century will be Ruled by the New Old*, New York: Tarcher.

Edmunds, J. and Turner, B.S. (2005) Global generations: Social change in the twentieth century, *British Journal of Sociology*, 56 (4): 559–77.

Elias, N. (1978) *The History of Manners. The Civilising Process; Volume I*, New York: Urizen Books.
—— (1985) *The Loneliness of Dying*, Oxford: Blackwell.
Elliott, A. and Lemert, C. (2006) *The New Individualism: The Emotional Costs of Globalisation*, London: Routledge.
Elliott, C. (2003) *Better than Well, American Medicine meets the American Dream*, London: W.W. Norton & Co.
Erikson, E. (1959) *Identity and the Life Cycle*, New York: International Universities Press.
Esping-Andersen, G. (1990) *The Three Worlds of Welfare Capitalism*, Cambridge: Polity Press.
—— (2000) The sustainability of welfare states into the twenty-first century, *International Journal of Health Services*, 30 (1): 1–12.
—— (Ed.) (2002) *Why we need a New Welfare State*, Oxford: Oxford University Press.
Estes, C.L. (1979) *The Aging Enterprise: A Critical Examination of Social Policies and Services for the Aged*, San Francisco: Jossey-Bass.
—— (2004) Social Security privatization and older women: A feminist political economy perspective, *Journal of Aging Studies*, 18 (1): 9–26.
—— (2001) *Social Policy and Aging: A Critical Perspective*, Thousand Oaks CA: Sage Publications.
Estes, C. and Mahakian, J. (2001) The political economy of productive aging, in N. Morrow-Howell, J. Hinterlong and M. Sherraden (Eds.) *Productive Aging: Concepts and Challenges*, 197–213, Baltimore MD: Johns Hopkins University Press.
Estes, C.L. and Phillipson, C. (2002) The globalization of capital, the welfare state, and old age policy, *International Journal of Health Services*, 32 (2): 279–97.
Estes, C., Biggs, S. and Phillipson, C. (2003) *Social Theory, Social Policy and Ageing: A Critical Introduction*, Maidenhead: Open University Press.
Estes, C.L., Linkins, K.W. and Binney, A. (1996) The political economy of aging, in R.H. Binstock and L.K. George (Eds.) *Handbook of Aging and the Social Sciences*, San Diego: Academic Press, 346–60.
European Commission (2000) *Social Policy Agenda, COM (2000)* Brussels, E.C.
Evandrou, M. (2005). Health and social care, in *Focus on Older People*, London: HMSO, 51–66.
Evandrou, M and Falkingham, J. (1993) Social security and the lifecourse: developing sensitive policy alternatives, in S. Arber and M. Evandrou (Eds.) *Ageing, Independence and the Lifecourse*, London: Jessica Kingsley, 201–23.
—— (2000) Looking back to look forward: lessons from four birth cohorts for ageing in the 21st Century, *Population Trends*, 99: 27–36.
Evans, J.G. (1997) Geriatric medicine a brief history, *British Medical Journal*, 315: 1075–78.
Fairclough, C. (2003) *Ageing bodies: Images and everyday experiences*, Walnut Creek: AltaMira Press.

Featherstone, M. (1991) Post-bodies, aging and virtual reality, in M. Featherstone and A. Wernick (Eds.) *Images of Aging, Cultural Representations of Later Life*, 227–44, London: Routledge.

Featherstone, M. and Hepworth, M. (1991) The mask of ageing and the post-modern lifecourse, in M. Featherstone, M. Hepworth and B.S. Turner (Eds.) *The Body: Social Processes and Cultural Theory*, London: Sage.

—— (1998), Ageing, the lifecourse and the sociology of embodiment, in G. Scambler and P. Higgs (Eds.) *Modernity, Medicine and Health*, London: Routledge.

Featherstone, M., Hepworth, M. and Turner, B.S. (Eds.) (1991) *The Body: Social Processes and Cultural Theory*, London: Sage.

Fitzpatrick, T. (2001) Making welfare for future generations, *Social Policy and Administration*, 35: 506–20.

Fogel, R. (1994) *The Relevance of Malthus for the Study of Mortality Today: Long-Run Influences on Health, Mortality, Labor Force Participation, and Population Growth*, NBER Working Paper 54, Washington DC: NBER.

Forrest, R. and Leather, P. (1998) The ageing of the property owning democracy, *Ageing and Society*, 18: 35–63.

Forth, C.E. and Crozier, I. (2005) *Body Parts, Critical Explorations in Corporeality*, New York: Lexington Books.

Foucault, M. (1973) *The Birth of the Clinic*, London: Tavistock.

—— (1977) *Discipline and Punish: the Birth of the Prison*, Harmondsworth: Penguin.

—— (1991) Governmentality, in Burchell, G., Gordon, C. and Miller, P. (Eds.) *The Foucault Effect: Studies in Governmentality*, Brighton: Harvester Wheatsheaf, 87–104.

Fox, N. (2002) Refracting 'health': Deleuze, Guattari and the body-self, *Health*, 6 (3): 347–63.

Fox, N.J. (1999) *Beyond Health: Postmodernism and Embodiment*, London: Free Association Books.

Fox, R.L. (2006) *The Classical World*, London: Penguin.

Franklin, S. (2007) *Dolly Mixtures: The Remaking of Geneology*, Durham NC: Duke University Press.

Freedman, M. (1999) *How Baby Boomers will Revolutionise Retirement and Transform America*, New York: Public Affairs.

Fries, J.F. (1980) Aging, natural death and the compression of morbidity, *New England Journal of Medicine*, 303: 130–35.

—— (1989) The compression of morbidity: near or far? *Millbank Quarterly*, 67: 208–32.

—— (2003) Measuring and monitoring success in compressing morbidity, *Annals of Internal Medicine*, 139: 455–59.

Gane, N. (2006) Posthuman, *Theory Culture and Society*, 23: 2–3, 431–34.

Garfinkel, H. (1967) *Studies in Ethnomethodology*, Englewood Cliffs, NJ: Prentice-Hall.

Garner, J.D. (Ed.) (1999) *Fundamentals of Feminist Gerontology*, New York: Haworth Press.

Gee, E. (2000) Population and politics: Voodoo demography, population aging and social policy, in E. Gee and G. Gutman (Eds.) *The Overselling of Population Aging: Apocalyptic Demography, Intergenerational Challenges and Social Policy*, 5–25, Don Mills, Ont: Oxford University Press.

Gerhardt, U. (1989) *Ideas about Illness: An Intellectual and Political History of Medical Sociology*, London: Macmillan.

Germov, J. (Ed.) (2005) *Second Opinion, an Introduction to Health Sociology*, 3rd Edition, Oxford: Oxford University Press.

Gershuny, J. (2000) *Changing Times: Work and Leisure in Post-industrial Society*, Oxford, Oxford University Press.

Giddens, A. (1990) *The Consequences of Modernity*, Cambridge, Polity Press.

—— (1991) *Modernity and Self-Identity. Self and Society in the Late Modern Age*, Cambridge: Polity Press.

—— (1994) Living in a post-traditional society, in U. Beck, A. Giddens and S. Lash, *Reflexive Modernization*, 56–109, Cambridge: Polity.

—— (1998) *The Third Way*, Cambridge: Polity.

—— (2000) *Runaway World: How Globalization Is Reshaping Our Lives*, London: Routledge.

Gilbert, N. (2002) *The Transformation of the Welfare State, The Silent Surrender of Public Responsibility*, Oxford: Oxford University Press.

Gilleard, C. (2002) Aging and old age in medieval society and the transition of modernity, *Journal of Aging and Identity*, 7: 25–41.

—— (2007) Old age in Byzantine society, *Ageing and Society*, 27: 623–42.

Gilleard, C. and Higgs, P. (1998) Older people as users and consumers of health care: A third age rhetoric for a fourth age reality, *Ageing and Society*, 18: 233–48.

—— (2000) *Cultures of Ageing: Self, Citizen and the Body*, Harlow: Pearson Education.

—— (2005) *Contexts of Ageing: Class, Cohort and Community*, Cambridge: Polity.

—— (2007a) Ageing without agency: Theorizing the fourth age. Finalist paper for 2007 GSA Social Gerontology Award, San Francisco, November 2007.

—— (2007b) The third age and the baby boomers: two approaches to the structuring of later life, *International Journal of Aging and Later Life*, 2 (2): 13–30.

Gilleard, C., Higgs, P., Hyde, M., Wiggins, R. and Blane, D. (2005b) Class, cohort and consumption: the British experience of the third age, *Journals of Gerontology: Social Sciences*, 60B: 305–10.

Gilligan, C. (1982) *In a Different Voice: Psychological Theory and Women's Development*, Cambridge: Harvard University Press.

Ginn, J. (2003) *Gender, Pensions and the Lifecourse*, Bristol: Policy Press.

Ginn, J. and Arber, S. (1995) Moving the goalposts: The impact on British women of raising their state pension age to 65, in J. Baldock and M. May (Eds.) *Social Policy Review No 7*, London: Social Policy Association, 1–20.

—— (2001) A colder pension climate for British women, in J. Ginn, D. Street and S. Arber (Eds.) *Women, Work and Pensions*, 44–66, Buckingham: Open University Press.

Glaser, B. and Strauss, A. (1968) *Time for Dying*, Chicago: University of Chicago Press.

Glaser, K., Murphy, M. and Grundy, E. (1997) Limiting long-term illness and household structure among people aged 45 and over, Great Britain 1991, *Ageing and Society*, 17:,3–19.

Goffman, E. (1959) *The Presentation of Self in Everyday Life*, New York: Anchor Books (Penguin edition 1990).

—— (1969) *The Presentation of Self in Everyday Life*, London: Penguin.

Goldsmith, M. (1996) *Hearing the Voice of People with Dementia: Opportunities and obstacles*. London: Jessica Kingsley Publishers.

Good, B. (1994) *Medicine, Rationality and Experience: An Anthropological Perspective*, Cambridge: Cambridge University Press.

Gough, I. (1979) *The Political Economy of the Welfare State*, London: Macmillan Press Ltd.

—— (2004) Human well-being and social structures: Relating the universal and the local, *Global Social Policy*, 4 (3): 289–311.

Government Actuary's Department (2007) *Lifetables*, www.gad.gov.uk/, downloaded 15 March 2007.

Graebner, W. (1980) *A History of Retirement: The Meaning and Function of an American Institution 1885–1978*, New Haven: Yale University Press.

Green, B.S. (1993) *Gerontology and the Construction of Old Age: A Study in Discourse Analysis*, New York: Aldine de Gruyter.

Greer, G. (1991) *The Change: Ageing and the Menopause*, Harmondsworth: Penguin.

Grosz, E. (1994) *Volatile Bodies: Toward a Corporeal Feminism (Theories of Representation and Difference)*, Sydney: Allen & Unwin.

—— (1995) *Space Time and Perversion, Essays on the Politics of Bodies*, London: Routledge.

Grundy, E. and Holt, G. (2001) The socioeconomic status of older adults: How should we measure it in studies of health inequalities? *Journal of Epidemiology and Community Health*, 55 (12): 895–904.

Grundy, E. and Sloggett, A. (2003) Health inequalities in the older population: the role of personal capital, social resources and socio-economic circumstances, *Social Science and Medicine*, 56: 935–47.

Gubrium, J. and Holstein, J. (2002) Going concerns and their bodies, in L. Anderson (ed.) *Cultural Gerontology*, 191–206, London: Auburn House.

Gullette, M.M. (2004) *Aged by Culture*, Chicago: University of Chicago Press.

Gustman, A.I. and Steinmeier, T.L. (2000) Pensions and retiree health benefits in household wealth: Changes from 1969 to 1992, *Journal of Human Resources*, 35 (1): 30–50.

Gutierrez-Robledo, L.M. (2002) Looking at the future of geriatric care in developing countries, *Journals of Gerontology Series, Biological Sciences and Medical Sciences*, 57 (2): M162–M167.

H.M. Treasury (2002) *Long-term Public Finance Report: An Analysis of Fiscal Sustainability*, London: H.M. Treasury.

Habermas, J. (2003) *The Future of Human Nature*, Cambridge: Polity.

Hagestad, G. and Dannefer, D. (2001) Concepts and theories of aging: beyond microfication in social science approaches, in R. Binstock and L. George (Eds.) *The Handbook of Aging*, 5th edn, San Diego: Academic Press.

HAI (1999) *The Ageing and Development Report: Poverty, Independence and the World's Older People*, Earthscan: London.

Hakim, C. (2000) *Work-lifestyle Choices in the 21st Century: Preference Theory*, Oxford: Oxford University Press.

—— (2007) Dancing with the devil? Essentialism and other feminist heresies, *British Journal of Sociology*, 58 (1): 123–32.

Haraway, D. (1991) *Simians, Cyborgs and Women: The Reinvention of Nature*, London: Routledge.

—— (1997) *Modest_Witness@Second_Millennium. FemaleMan©_ Meets_Onco Mouse^TM*, London: Routledge.

Harper, S. (2006) *Ageing Societies: Myths, Challenges and Opportunities*, London: Hodder Arnold.

Harper, S. and Thane, P. (1989) The consolidation of 'old age' as a phase of life 1945–65, in M. Jefferys (Ed.) *Growing Old in the Twentieth Century*, 41–61, London: Routledge.

Harvey, D. (1996) *Justice, Nature and the Geography of Difference*, Oxford: Blackwell.

—— (2005) *A Brief History of Neoliberalism*, Oxford: Oxford University Press.

Heinz, W.R. (1996) Status passages as micro-macro linkages in life course research, in A. Weymann and W.R. Heinz (Eds.) *Society and Biography: Interrelationships between Social Structure, Institutions and the Life Course*, Weinheim: Deutscher Studien Verlag.

Held, D. (2004) *Global Covenant, The Social Democratic Alternative to the Washington Consensus*, Cambridge: Polity.

Held, D., McGrew, A., Goldblatt, D. and Perraton, J. (1999) *Global Transformations: Politics, Economics and Culture*, Cambridge: Polity Press.

HelpAge International (2002) *State of the World's Older People, 2002*, London: HelpAge International.

Hepworth, M. (1988) Ageing and the emotions, in G. Bendelow and S.J. Williams (Eds.) *Emotions in Social Life: Critical Themes and Contemporary Issues*, 56–68, London: Routledge.

Higgs, P., Hyde, M., Wiggins, R. and Blane, D. (2003) Researching quality of life in early old age: The importance of the sociological dimension, *Social Policy and Administration*, 37: 239–52.

Higgs, P. and Jones, I.R. (2003) Ultra-Darwinism and Health: the limits to evolutionary psychology, in S. Williams, L. Burke and G. Bendelow (Eds.) *Debating Biology: Sociological Reflections on Health, Medicine and Society*, 27–38, London: Routledge.

Higgs, P. and Gilleard, C. (2006) Departing the margins: Social class and later life in a second modernity, *Journal of Sociology*, 42: 219–41.

Higgs, P., Evandrou, M., Gilleard, C., Hyde, M., Jones, I.R., Victor, C. and Wiggins, D. (2007) Ageing and consumption patterns in Britain, 1968–2001, *Generations Review*, 17: 1.

Hill, M. (2007) *Pensions*, Bristol: Policy Press.

Hills, J. (2004) *Inequality and the State*, Oxford: Oxford University Press.

Hilton, C. (2005) The origins of old age psychiatry in Britain in the 1940s, *History of Psychiatry*, 16 (3): 267–89.

Hinterlong, J., Morrow-Howell, N. and Sherraden, M. (2001) Productive aging: Principles and perspectives, in N. Morrow-Howell, J. Hinterlong and M. Sherraden (Eds.) *Productive Aging: Concepts and Challenges*, Baltimore MD: Johns Hopkins University Press, 3–18.

Hochschild, A.R. (1975) Disengagement theory: A critique and proposal, *American Sociological Review*, 40: 553–69.

Hockey, J. and James, A. (1993) *Growing Up and Growing Old: Ageing and Dependency in the Life Course*, London: Sage.

Hogle, L.F. (2005) Enhancement technologies and the body, *Annual Review of Anthropology*, 34: 695–716.

Holmes, E. and Holmes, L. (1995) *Other Cultures, Elder Years*, Thousand Oaks: Sage.

Holstein, M. (1999) Women and productive aging: Troubling implications, in M. Minkler and C. Estes (Eds.) *Critical Gerontology*, Amityville, NY: Baywood.

Holstein, M. and Minkler, M. (Eds.) (2003) Self, society and the new gerontology, *Gerontologist*, 43 (6): 787–96.

House of Lords (2005) *Lords Science and Technology Committee, 1st Report, 21st July 2005, Volume I*, HL Paper No 20-I, London: House of Lords.

Hughes, B. and Paterson, K. (1997) The social model of disability and the disappearing body: towards a sociology of impairment, *Disability and Society*, 12 (3): 325–40.

Hunt, K. (2002) A generation apart? Gender-related experiences and health in women in early and late mid-life, *Social Science and Medicine*, 54: 663–76.

Hyde, M. and Jones, I.R. (2007) The long shadow of work? Does time since labour market exit affect the association between socio-economic position and health in a post working population? *Journal of Epidemiology and Community Health*, 61 (6): 532–38.

Illich, I. (1976) *Limits to Medicine: Medical Nemesis: The Expropriation of Health*, Harmondsworth: Pelican.

Jappelli, T. (1999) The age-wealth profile and the life-cycle hypothesis: a cohort analysis with a time series of cross-sections of Italian households, *Review of Income and Wealth*, 45: 57–76.

Jeffreys, M. (1991) Medical sociology and public health: Interdisciplinary Rrelationships 1950–90, *Public Health*, 105: 15–21.

—— (1997) Social medicine and medical sociology 1950–70, The testimony of a partisan participant, in D. Porter, (Ed.) *Social Medicine and Medical Sociology in the Twentieth Century*, Amsterdam: Rodopi, B. V.

Jeffreys, S. (2005) *Beauty and Misogyny: Harmful Practices in the West*, London: Routledge.

Jones, I.R., Hyde, M., Victor, C., Wiggins, R., Gilleard, C. and Higgs, P. (2008) *Ageing in a Consumer Society: From Passive to Active Consumption in Britain*, Bristol: Policy Press.

Juengst, E., Binstock, R., Mehlman, M., Post, S. and Whitehouse, P. (2003) Biogerontology, 'anti-aging medicine', and the challenges of human enhancement, *Hastings Center Report*, 33 (4): 21–30.

Katz, S. (1996) *Disciplining Old Age: The Formation of Gerontological Knowledge*, London: University Press of Virginia.

—— (2005) *Cultural Aging: Lifecourse, lifestyle and Senior Worlds*, Peterborough Ont.: Broadview Press.

Katz, S. and Marshall, B. (2003) New sex for old: lifestyle, consumerism, and the ethics of aging well, *Journal of Aging Studies*, 17: 3–16.

Kelly, M. and Field, D. (1996) Medical sociology, chronic illness and the body, *Sociology of Health and Illness*, 18 (2): 241–57.

King, C. (2003) Imagining the third age: symbolic exchange and old age, *Health Sociology Review*, 12: 156–62.

King, R., Warnes, A. and Williams, A. (1998) International retirement migration in Europe, *International Journal of Population Geography*, 4: 91–112.

Kirkwood, T. (1999) *Time of our Lives: The Science of Human Ageing*, London: Weidenfeld & Nicolson.

—— (2001) *The End of Age*, London: Profile Books.

—— (2004) Review of Benecke: The Dream of Eternal Life, *Ageing and Society*, 24 (3): 482–84.

Kitwood, T. (1997) *Dementia reconsidered: The person comes first*, Buckingham: Open University Press.

Kitwood, T. and Benson, S. (Eds.) (1995) *The New Culture of Dementia Care*, London: Hawker Publications.

Klatz, R. (1996) *Advances in Anti-Aging Medicine Volume 1*, NewYork: Mary Ann Liebert Inc.

Kontos, P. (1999) Local biology: Bodies of difference in ageing studies, *Ageing and Society*, 19: 677–89.

Kotlikoff, L.J. (2003) *Generational Policy*, Cambridge, MA: MIT Press.

Land, K.C. and Russell, S.T. (1996) Wealth Accumulation across the adult life course: Stability and change in sociodemographic covariate structures of net worth data in the survey of income and program participation, 1984–91, *Social Science Research*, 25 (4): 423–62.

Lash, S. and Urry, J. (1987) *The End of Organized Capitalism*, Cambridge: Polity Press.

—— (1996) *The End of Organized Capitalism*, Cambridge: Polity Press.

Laslett, P. (1996, 1989) *A Fresh Map of Life, The Emergence of the Third Age*, 2nd edition, Basingstoke: Macmillan Press Ltd.

Latour, B. (2003) Is *re*-modernization occurring – and if so, how to prove it? *Theory Culture and Society*, 20 (2): 35–48.

Lawler, J. (1997) (Ed.) *The Body in Nursing*, Melbourne: Churchill Livingstone.

Lawson, T. (2003) *Reorienting Economics*, London: Routledge.

Lawton, J. (1998) Contemporary hospice care: the sequestration of the unbounded body and 'dirty dying', *Sociology of Health and Illness*, 20 (2): 121–43.

—— (2000) *The Dying Process: Patients' Experiences of Palliative Care*, London: Routledge.

Leon, D. and McCambridge, J. (2006) Liver cirrhosis mortality rates in Britain from 1950–2002: an analysis of routine data, *Lancet*, 367: 52–56.

Levy, R. (1996) Toward a theory of life course institutionalization, in A. Weymann and W.R. Heinz (Eds.) *Society and Biography: Interrelationships between Social Structure, Institutions and the Life Course*, Weinheim: Deutscher Studien Verlag.

Lewis, J. (2007) Gender, agency and the 'new social settlement', the importance of developing a holistic approach to care policies, *Current Sociology*, 55 (2): 271–86.

Lewis, M. and Butler, R. (1972) Why is Women's Lib ignoring old women, *International Journal of Aging: Human Development*, 3: 223–31.

Lippman, A. (1992) Led (astray) by genetic maps: the cartography of the human genome and health care, *Social Science and Medicine*, 25 (12): 1469–76.

Lloyd, L. (2004) Mortality and morality: ageing and the ethics of care, *Ageing and Society*, 24: 235–56.

Lock, M. (1993) *Encounters with aging: mythologies of menopause in Japan and North America*, Berkeley CA: University of California Press.

Longino, C. (1988) The gray peril mentality and the impact of retirement migration, *Journal of Appied Gerontology*, 7: 448–55.

Lords Science and Technology Committee (2005), *First Report*, 21st July 2005.

—— (2006), *Sixth Report*, 14th March 2006.

Luborsky, M.R. (1994) The retirement process – making the person and cultural meanings malleable, *Medical Anthropology Quarterly*, 8 (4): 411–29.

Lupton, D. (1995) *The Imperative of Health, Public Health and the Regulated Body*, London: Sage.

—— (1997) Consumerism, reflexivity and the medical encounter, *Social Science and Medicine*, 45: 373–81.

Macintyre, S., Hunt, K. and Sweeting, H. (1996) Gender differences in health, are things really as simple as they seem? *Social Science and Medicine*, 42: 617–24.

Manton, K.G. (1982) Changing concepts of morbidity and mortality in the elderly population, *Milbank Memorial Fund Quarterly – Health and Society*, 60(2): 183–244.

Manton, K.G. and Gu, X. (2001) Changes in the prevalence of chronic disability in the United States black and nonblack population above age 65 from 1982 to 1999, *Proceedings of the National Academy of Science*, 98: 6354–59.

Marshall, B. (2002) Forever functional: sexual fitness and the ageing male body, *Body and Society*, 8 (4): 43–70.

Martin, E. (2000) Mind-body problems, *American Ethnologist*, 27 (3): 569–90.

McKee, K.J. (1999) The body drop – age and recovery from disabling events, *Proceedings of the British Psychological Society*, 7: 19.

McMunn, A., Breeze, E., Goodman, A., Nazroo, J. and Oldfield, Z. (2006) Social determinants of health in older age, in M. Marmot and R.G. Wilkinson, *Social Determinants of Health*, 2nd edition, Oxford: Oxford University Press.

McNicol, J. and Blaikie, A. (1989) The politics of retirement 1908–48, in M. Jefferys (Ed.) *Growing Old in the Twentieth Century*, London: Routledge, 21–42.

Medina, J. (1996) *The Clock of Ages: Why we age, How we age, Winding Back the Clock*, Cambridge: Cambridge University Press.

Mellor, P. (1993) Death in high modernity, in D. Clarke (Ed.) *The Sociology of Death*, Oxford: Blackwell.

Mellor, P. and Shilling, P. (1993) Modernity, self-identity and the sequestration of death, *Sociology*, 27 (3): 411–31.

Melzer, D. (1998) New drug treatment for Alzheimer's disease: lessons for healthcare policy, *British Medical Journal*, 316: 762–64.

Merleau-Ponty, M. (2002 [1962]) *Phenomenology of Perception*, London: Routledge.

Midwinter, E. (2005) How many people are there in the third age? *Ageing and Society*, 25: 9–18.

Minkler, M. and Estes, C. (eds.) *Critical Gerontology: Perspectives from Political and Moral Economy*, Amityville, NY: Baywood.

Minns, R. (2001) *The Cold War in Welfare: Stock Markets Versus Pensions*, London: Verso.

—— (2006) *The future of stock market pensions*, in J.A. Vincent, C.R. Phillipson and M. Downs (Eds.) *The Futures of Old Age*, 98–106, London: Sage.

Mishra, R. (1999) *Globalization and the Welfare State*, Cheltenham: Edward Elgar.

Moody, H.R. (1993) Overview: What is critical gerontology and why is it important? in T.R. Cole, W.A. Achenbaum, P.L. Jakobi and R. Kastenbaum (Eds.) *Voices and Visions of Aging: Toward a Critical Gerontology*, New York: Springer.

—— (1995) Ageing, meaning and the allocation of resources, *Ageing and Society*, 15: 163–84.

—— (2002) Who's afraid of life extension? *Generations*, special edition on Anti-Aging: Are You For It Or Against It? 25 (4): 33–37.

Morris, G., Cook, D. and Shaper, A. (1994) Loss of employment and mortality, *British Medical Journal*, 308: 1135–39.

Murphy, J. and Longino, C. (1997) Toward a postmodern understanding of aging and identity, *Journal of Aging and Identity*, 2 (2): 81–89.

Mykytyn, C. (2006) Anti-aging medicine: a patient/practitioner movement to redefine aging, *Social Science and Medicine*, 62: 643–53.

Myles, J. (1989) *Old Age in the Welfare State: The Political Economy of Public Pensions*, University Press of Kansas.

—— (2002) A new contract for the elderly? in G. Esping-Andersen (Ed.) *Why we need a New Welfare State*, 130–72, Oxford: Oxford University Press.

Naess, O., Hernes, F.H. and Blane, D. (2006). Life-course influences on mortality at older ages: Evidence from the Oslo Mortality Study, *Social Science and Medicine*, 62: 329–36.

Nettleton, S. (2007) *The Sociology of Health and Illness*, 2nd edition, Cambridge: Polity Press.

Neugarten, B.L. (1974) Age-groups in American society and the rise of the young-old, *Annals of the American Academy of Politics and Social Sciences*, 9: 187–98.

—— (1996) *The Meanings of Age: Selected Papers of Bernice L. Neugarten*, Chicago: Chicago University Press.

Neugarten, B.L. and Associates. (1964) *Personality in Middle and Later Life*, New York: Atherton.

Newton, T. (2003) Crossing the great divide: Time, nature and the social, *Sociology*, 37: 433–57.

Novas, C. and Rose, N. (2000) Genetic risk and the birth of the somatic individual, *Economy and Society*, 29 (4): 485–513.

O'Rand, A. and Krecker, M. (1990) Concepts of the life cycle: Their history, meanings and uses in the social sciences, *Annual Review of Sociology*, 16: 241–62.

O'Sullivan, M. (2000) Corporate governance and globalization, *Annals of the American Academy of Political and Social Sciences*, 570: 153–72.

Offe, C. (1985) *Disorganized Capitalism*, Cambridge: Polity Press.

Oliver, M. (1996) *Understanding Disability: From Theory to Practice*, London: Macmillan.

Olshansky, S.J., Carnes, B.A. and Grahn, D. (1998) Confronting the boundaries of human longevity, *American Scientist*, 86: 52–61.

Olshansky, S.J., Carnes, B.A. and Désesquelles, A. (2001) Prospects for longevity, *Science*, 291: 1491–92.

Olshansky, S., Hayflick, L. and Carnes, B.(2002) No truth to the Fountain of Youth, *Scientific American*, 286: 78–81.

Olshansky, S.J., Passaro, D.I., Hershaw, R.C., Layden, J., Carnes, B.A., Broody, J., Hayflick, L., Bulter, R.N., Allinson, D.B. and Ludwig, D.S. (2005) A potential decline in life expectancy in the United States in the 21st century, *New England Journal of Medicine*, 352: 1138–45.

Omran, A.R. (2005) The epidemiologic transition: A theory of the epidemiology of population change, *Milbank Quarterly*, 83 (4): 731–57.

ONS (2004) *Healthy Life Expectancies for Great Britain and England: Annual estimates 1981–2001*, www.statistics.gov.uk/downloads/theme_health/Healthy_Life_Expectancy.pdf accessed 10th April 2008.

Outhwaite, W. (2006) *The Future of Society*, London: Blackwell.

Pahl, J. (2005) Individualization in couple finances: who pays for the children? *Social Policy and Society*, 4: 381–91.

Palacios, R. (2002) The future of global ageing, *International Journal of Epidemiology*, 31: 786–91.

Parker, M.G. and Thorslund, M. (2007) Health trends in the elderly population: Getting better and getting worse, *Gerontologist*, 47 (2): 150–58.

Parsons, T. (1942) Age and sex in the social structure of the United States, *American Sociological Review*, 7: 604–616.

——(1951) *The Social System*, London: Routledge and Kegan Paul.

Pensions Commission (2005) *A New Pension Settlement for the Twenty-First Century, The Second Report of the Pensions Commission*, London: The Stationery Office.

Peracchi, F. and Welch, F. (1994). Trends in labor force transitions of older men and women, *Journal of Labor Economics*, 12 (2): 210–42.

Phillips, J. (2007) *Care*, Cambridge: Polity Press.

Phillipson, C. (1982) *Capitalism and the Construction of Old Age*, London: Macmillan.

—— (1998) *Reconstructing Old Age, New Agendas in Social Theory and Practice*, London: Sage.

—— (2003) Globalisation and the future of ageing: Developing a critical gerontology, *Sociological Research Online*, 8 (4): 1–13. www.socresonline.org.uk/8/4/philliposn.html, accessed December 2004.

—— (2006) Ageing and globalisation, in Vincent, C., Phillipson, C. and Downs, M. (Eds.) *The Future of Old Age*, 201–7, London: Sage.

Phillipson, C. and Baars, J. (2007) Social theory and social ageing, in J. Bond, S. Peace, F. Dittmann-Kohli and G. Westerhof, (Eds.) *Ageing in Society*, 3rd Edition, London: Sage.

Phillipson, C., Baars, J., Dannefer, D. and Walker, A. (Eds.) (2006) *Aging, Globalisation and Inequality: The New Critical Gerontology*, New York: Baywood Press.

Pitts, V. (2003) *In the Flesh: The Cultural Politics of Body Modification*, New York: Palgrave.

Polivka, L. (2000) Postmodern aging and the loss of meaning, *Journal of Aging and Identity*, 5 (4): 225–35.

—— (2001) Globalization, population, aging and ethics, *Journal of Aging and Identity*, 6: 147–63.

Post, S. and Binstock, R. (Eds.) (2004) *Fountain of Youth: Cultural, Scientific and Ethical Perspectives on a Biomedical Goal*, Oxford: Oxford University Press.

Pound, P., Bury, M., Gompertz, P. and Ebrahim, S. (1995) Stroke patients' views on their admission to hospital, *BMJ*, 311: 18–22.

Powell, J.L. and Biggs, S. (2000) Managing old age: The disciplinary web of power, surveillance and normalisation, *Journal of Aging and Identity*, 5 (1): 3–13.

Powell, J.L. and Longino, C.F. (2001) Towards the postmodernization of aging: The body and social theory, *Journal of Aging and Identity*, 6 (4): 199–207.

Price, D. and Ginn, J. (2006) The future of inequalities in retirement income, in J.A. Vincent, C.R. Phillipson and M. Downs (Eds.) *The Futures of Old Age*, London: Sage.

Putnam, R. D. (2000) *Bowling Alone: The Collapse and Revival of American Community*, New York: Simon & Schuster.

Quaade, T., Engholm, G., Johansen, A.M.T. and Moller, H. (2002) Mortality in relation to early retirement in Denmark: a population-based study, *Scandinavian Journal of Public Health*, 30 (3): 216–22.

Quadagno, J., Hardy, M. and Hazelrigg, L. (2003) Labour market transitions and the erosion of the Fordist lifecycle: Discarding older workers in the automobile manufacturing and banking industries in the United States, *Geneva Papers on Risk and Insurance – Issues and Practice*, 28 (4): 640–51.

Rabinow, P. (Ed.) (1984) *The Foucault Reader*, London: Penguin Books.

Ramsay, S.E., Morris, R.W., Lennon, L.T., Wannamethee, S.G. and Whincup, P. H. (2008) Are social inequalities in mortality in Britain narrowing? Time trends from 1978 to 2005 in a population-based study of older men, *Journal of Epidemiology Community Health*, 62: 75–80.

Ransome, P. (2005) *Work, Consumption and Culture: Affluence and Social Change in the Twenty First Century*, London: Sage.

Ray, R.E. (1999) Researching to transgress: The need for critical feminism in gerontology, *Journal of Women and Aging*, 11 (2/3): 171–84.

—— (2004) Toward the croning of feminist gerontology, *Journal of Aging Studies*, 18 (1): 1109–21.

Rigg, J. and Sefton, T. (2006) Income dynamics and the life cycle, *Journal of Social Policy*, 35: 411–35.

Riley, M.W., Johnson, M. and Foner, A. (1972) *Aging and Society, Volume III: A Sociology of Age*, New York: Russell Sage Foundation.

Rose, H. and Rose, S. (2001) (Eds.) *Alas Poor Darwin, Arguments Against Evolutionary Psychology*, London: Vintage.

Rose, N. (2001) The politics of life itself, *Theory, Culture and Society*, 18 (6): 1–30.

—— (2007a) Molecular biopolitics, somatic ethics and the spirit of biocapital, *Social Theory and Health*, 5: 3–29.

—— (2007b) *The Politics of Life Itself: Biomedicine, Power and Subjectivity in the Twenty-First Century*, Princeton NJ: Princeton University Press.

Rowe, J.W. and Kahn, R.C. (1987) Human ageing: Usual and successful, *Science*, 237: 143–49.

—— (1998) *Successful Aging*, New York: Pantheon.

Rowntree, B.S. (1901) *Poverty: A Study of Town Life*, Macmillan: London.

—— (1947) *Poverty and Progress: A Second Social Survey of York*, London: Longmans.

Ruhm, C.J. (1995) Secular changes in the work and retirement patterns of older men, *Journal of Human Resources*, 30 (2): 362–85.

Sanders, C., Donovan, J.L. and Dieppe, P.A. (2002) The significance and consequences of having painful and disabled joints in older age: coexisting accounts of normal and disrupted biographies, *Sociology of Health and Illness*, 24: 227–253.

Sassatelli, R. (2007) *Consumer Culture: History, Theory and Politics*, London: Sage.

Sauvy, A. (1947) Social and economic consequences of the ageing of Western European populations, *Population Studies*, 2: 115–4.

Savage, M. (2000) *Class Analysis and Social Transformation*, Buckingham: Open University Press.

Savage, M., Bagnall, G. and Longhurst, B.L. (2001) Ordinary, ambivalent and defensive: class identities in the North-West of England, *Sociology*, 35: 875–92.

Sayer, A. (2000) *Realism and Social Science*, London: Sage.

Scambler, G. (2002) *Health and Social Change: A Critical Theory*, Buckingham: Open University Press.

Schilling, O.K. (2005) Cohort and age-related decline in elders' life satisfaction: is there really a paradox? *European Journal of Ageing*, 2: 254–63.

Schoeni, R.F., Freedman, V.A. and Martin, L.G. (2008) Why is late-life disability declining? *The Milbank Quarterly*, 86 (1): 47–89.

Scourfield, P. (2007) Are there reasons to be worried about the 'caretelization' of residential care? *Critical Social Policy*, 27: 155–80.

Seccombe, W. (1993) *Weathering the Storm, Working-Class Families from the Industrial Revolution to the Fertility Decline*, London: Verso.

Seidman, S. (1997) *Difference Troubles: Queering Social Theory and Sexual Politics*, Cambridge: Cambridge University Press.

Sennett, R. (1994) *Flesh and Stone, The Body and the City in Western Civilization*, London: Faber and Faber.

—— (1998) *The Corrosion of Character*, New York: W. W. Norton & Co.

—— (2006) *The Culture of the New Capitalism*, New Haven: Yale University Press.

Settersen, R. (1998) Time, age and transition to retirement: New evidence on life course flexibility, *International Journal of Aging and Human Development*, 47: 177–203.

Shilling, C. (1993) *The Body and Social Theory*, London: Sage.

—— (1997) The body and difference, in Woodward K. (Ed.) *Identity and Difference* (Ch. 2) London: Sage/Open University, 63–121.

—— (2005) *The Body in Culture, Technology and Society*, London: Sage.

Shuey, K. and O'Rand, A. (2006) Changing demographics and new pension risks, *Research on Aging*, 28: 317–40.

Silver, C.B. (2003) Gendered identities in old age: Toward (de)gendering? *Journal of Aging Studies*, 17 (4): 379–97.

Singh, C. and Kelly, M. (2003) Botox: an 'elixir of youth'? *European Journal of Plastic Surgery*, 26 (5): 273–74.

Smart, B. (1993) *Postmodernity*, London: Routledge.

Smith, J. (2001) Well-being and health from age 70 to 100: findings from the Berlin Ageing Study, *European Review*, 9 (4): 461–77.

Smith, J. and Baltes, P.B. (1999) Trends and profiles of psychological functioning in very old age, in P.B. Baltes and K.U. Mayer (Eds.) *The Berlin Ageing Study: Ageing from 70 to 100*, Cambridge: Cambridge University Press.

Sontag, S. (1989) *Illness as a Metaphor/AIDS and its Metaphors*, New York: Anchor.

Soper, K. (1995) *What is Nature?* Oxford: Blackwell.

SOSTRIS (1999) *Working Paper 9: The Final Report*, London, Centre for Biography in Social Policy: University of East London.

Strauss, R. (1957) The nature and status of medical sociology, *American Sociological Review*, 22: 200–204.

Sudnow, D. (1967) *Passing on: The Social Organisation of Dying*, Englewood Cliffs, New Jersey: Prentice Hall.

Sulkunen, P. (1997) Introduction in P. Sulkunen, J. Holmwood, H. Radner and G. Shulze (Eds.) *Constructing the New Consumer Society*, London: Macmillan.

Suzman, R.M., Willis, D.P. and Manton, K.G. (Eds.) (1992) *The Oldest Old*, Oxford: Oxford University Press.

Tallis, R. (2005) Living longer, healthier lives, *The Times*, 22 October 2005.

Taylor, P.E. and Walker, A. (1994) The aging workforce – employers attitudes towards older-people, *Work Employment and Society*, 8 (4): 569–91.

Taylor-Gooby, P. (2002) The Silver age of the welfare state: perspectives on resilience, *Journal of Social Policy*, 31: 597–621.

Thane, P. (2003) Social histories of old age and aging, *Journal of Social History*, 37 (1): 93–111.

The Death Clock (2007) www.deathclock.com/ accessed 15 May 2007.

Thomas, C. (2007) *Sociologies of Disability and Illness: Contested Ideas in Disability Studies and Medical Sociology*, London: Palgrave.

Thomson, D. (1989) The welfare state and generational conflict: winners and losers, in P. Johnson, C. Conrad and D. Thomson (Eds.) *Workers Versus Pensioners: Intergenerational Justice in an Ageing World*, Manchester: Manchester University Press, 33–56.

Tilly, C. and Tilly, C. (1998) *Work under Capitalism*, Westview Press: Colorado.

Townsend, P. (1957) *The Family Life of Old People: An Inquiry in East London*, London: Routledge and Kegan Paul.

—— (1963) *The Last Refuge, A Survey of Residential Institutions and Homes for the Aged in England and Wales*, London: Routledge and Kegan Paul.

—— (1981) The structured dependency of the elderly: the creation of social policy in the 20th century, *Ageing and Society*, 1: 5–28.

—— (1986) Ageism and social policy, in C. Phillipson and A. Walker (Eds.) *Ageing and Social Policy: A Critical Assessment*, 15–44, Aldershot: Gower.

Townsend, P. and Walker, A. (1995) *New Directions for Pensions: How to Revitalise National Insurance Pamphlet No 2*, Nottingham: European Labour Forum.

Tretheway, M. and Mak, D. (2005) Emerging tourist markets: Ageing and developing economies, *Journal of Air Transport Management*, 12: 21–27.

Tsai, S.P., Wendt, J.K., Donnelly, R.P., de Jong, G. and Ahmed, F.S. (2005) Age at retirement and long-term survival of an industrial population: prospective cohort study, *British Medical Journal*, 331 (7523): 995–97.

Tulle, E. (2007) Running to run: Embodiment, structure and agency amongst veteran elite runners, *Sociology*, 41 (2): 329–46.

Turner, B.S. (1987) *Medical Power and Social Knowledge*, London: Sage.

—— (1989) Ageing, status politics and sociological theory, *The British Journal of Sociology*, 40 (4): 588–606.

—— (1995) Aging and identity: Some reflections on the somatization of the self, in M. Featherstone and A. Wernick (Eds.) *Images of Aging: Cultural Representations of Later Life*, London: Routledge.

—— (1996) *The Body and Society*, London: Sage.

—— (1998) Ageing and generational conflicts: a reply to Sarah Irwin, *The British Journal of Sociology*, 49: 299–304.

—— (2000) The history of the changing concept of health and illness: outline of a general model of illness categories, in G.L. Albrecht, R. Fitzpatrick and S.C. Scrimshaw, *The Handbook of Social Studies in Health and Medicine*, 9–23, London: Sage.

—— (2004) *The New Medical Sociology: Social Forms of Health and Illness*, New York: W.W. Norton.

—— (2006) Classical sociology and cosmopolitanism: a critical defence of the social, *The British Journal of Sociology*, 57 (1): 133–52.

Twigg, J. (2000) Carework as bodywork, *Ageing and Society*, (20): 389–411.

—— (2002) The Body in Social Policy: Mapping a Territory, *Journal of Social Policy*, 31 (3): 421–39.

—— (2004) The body, gender and age: Feminist insights in social gerontology, *Journal of Ageing Studies*, 18: 59–73.

—— (2006) *The Body in Health and Social Care*, London: Palgrave.

—— (2007) Clothing, age and the body, *Ageing and Society*, 27, 2007: 285–305

United Nations (2002) *World Population Ageing: 1950–2050*, Department of Economic and Social Affairs Population Division, New York: United Nations.

Vågero, D. (1996) European medical sociology: a comment on Margot Jeffreys' view, *European Journal of Public Health*, 6 (2): 98–99.

Vickerstaff, S. and Cox, J. (2005) Retirement and risk: the individualisation of retirement experiences? *Sociological Review*, 53 (1): 77–95.

Victor, C. (1994) *Old Age in Modern Society*, London: Chapman and Hall.

—— (2006) Will old age be healthier? in J. Vincent, M. Downs and C. Phillipson (Eds.) *The Future of Old Age*, 138–46, London: Sage.

Vincent, J. (1999), *Politics, Power and Old Age*, Buckingham: Open University Press.

—— (2003a) *Old Age*, London: Routledge.

—— (2003b) What is at stake in the 'War on anti-ageing medicine'? *Ageing and Society*, 23: 675–84.

—— (2006a) Anti-ageing science and the future of old age, in Vincent, C., Phillipson, C. and Downs, M. (Eds.) *The Future of Old Age*, 192–200, London: Sage.

—— (2006b) Ageing contested: anti-ageing science and the cultural construction of old age, *Sociology*, 40: 681–98.

Wadsworth, M.E.J. (1991) *The Imprint of Time; Childhood, History and Adult life*, Oxford: Oxford University Press.

Wainwright, S.P. and Turner, B.S. (2006) 'Just crumbling to bits'? An exploration of the body, ageing, injury and career in classical ballet dancers, *Sociology*, 40: 237–55.

Walker, A. (1981) Towards a political economy of old age, *Ageing and Society*, 1 (1): 73–94.

—— (2005) Towards an international political economy of ageing, *Ageing and Society*, 25: 815–39.

Walker, B.G. (1985) *The Crone: Woman of Age, Wisdom and Power*, New York: Harper Collins.

Wanless, D. (2001) *Securing our Future Health: Taking a Long-term View*, London: H.M. Treasury.

Warnes, T. (2006) The future life course, migration and old age, in J.A. Vincent, C.R. Phillipson and M. Downs (Eds.) *The Futures of Old Age*, 208–17, London: Sage.

Warren, M. (1943) Care of chronic sick: a case for treating chronic sick in blocks in a general hospital, *British Medical Journal*, ii, 822–23.

Weagley, R.O. and Huh, E. (2004a) Leisure expenditures of retired and near-retired households, *Journal of Leisure Research*, 36 (1): 101–27.

—— (2004b) The impact of retirement on household leisure expenditures, *Journal of Consumer Affairs*, 38 (2): 262–81.

Webster, C. and Rice, S. (1996) Equity theory and the power structure in a marital relationship, *Advances in Consumer Research*, 23 (23): 491–97.

Weiss, R.S. and Bass, S.A. (Eds.) (2001) *Challenges of the Third Age, Meaning and Purpose in Later Life*, 3–12, Oxford: Oxford University Press.

Wiatrowski, W.J. (2001) Changing retirement age: Ups and downs, *Monthly Labor Review*, 124.

Williams, G. (1984) The genesis of chronic illness: narrative reconstruction, *Sociology of Health and Illness*, 6: 175–200.

—— (2000) Knowledgeable narratives, *Anthropology and Medicine*, 7 (1): 135–40.

—— (2003) The determinants of health: structure context and agency, *Sociology of Health and Illness*, 25: 131–54.

Williams, S. (1993) *Chronic Respiratory Illness* London: Routledge.

Williams, S.J. (2000) Chronic illness as biographical disruption or biographical disruption as chronic illness? Reflections on a core concept, *Sociology of Health and Illness*, 22 (1): 40–67.

—— (2003) *Medicine and the Body*, London: Sage.

—— (2004) Beyond medicalization-healthicization? A rejoinder to Hislop and Arber, *Sociology of Health and Illness*, 26 (4): 453–59.

Williams, S.J. and Bendelow, G. (1998) *The Lived Body: Sociological Themes, Embodied Issues*, London: Routledge.

Wilson, G. (1997) A postmodern approach to structured dependency theory, *Journal of Social Policy*, 26: 341–50.

Wilson, A.E., Shuey, K.M. and Elder, G.H. (2007) Cumulative advantage processes as mechanisms of inequality in life course health, *American Journal of Sociology*, 112 (6): 1886–1924.

Wister, A.N. (2005) *Baby Boomer Health Dynamics, How are we Ageing*, Toronto: University of Toronto Press.

Woodward, K. (1991) *Aging and Its Discontents: Freud and Other Fictions*, Bloomington: Indiana University Press.

World Bank (1994) *Averting the Old Age Crisis*, Oxford: Oxford University Press.

—— (2005) *Old-Age Income Support in the 21st Century: An International Perspective on Pension Systems and Reform*, Washington: The World Bank.

Zaidi, A., Frick, J.R. and Buchel, F. (2005) Income mobility in old age in Britain and Germany, *Ageing and Society*, 25: 543–65.

Zarb, G. and Oliver, M. (1993) *Ageing with a Disability: What Do They Expect After All These Years?* London: University of Greenwich.

Ziguras, C. (2004) *Self-Care: Embodiment, Personal Autonomy and the Shaping of Health Consciousness*, Routledge: London.

Zola, I.K. (1970) Medicine as an institution of social control: the medicalizing of society, *Sociological Review*, 20 (4): 487–504.

Index

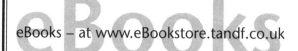